The food anthropologist

... a one year journey revisited

H. Sofia de Campos Pereira

The Food Anthropologist

To my homies, Patrick, Sara and Tomas, for encouraging me to fly while keeping me anchored.

The Food Anthropologist

CONTENTS

H. Sofia de Campos Pereira

Acknowledgements

This book narrates my incredible one-year long experiment through consecutive food challenges, a journey that would have been impossible without the support and encouragement of many. First of all, my clients, who trust me and constantly inspire me to become the best health coach that I can be. Thanks to you, I sought to go further in my food journey as well as to learn more about nutrition theory. In the end, I am a better health coach because of this experience.

I am also grateful to all my friends and family. To those that stayed engaged through my consecutive limitations and experiments, personally or on social media, thank you for your input, encouragement, and humor. If you had the misfortune of sitting at a table and sharing a meal with me throughout the year of challenges, I thank you for your patience and understanding, especially if I ate only a small portion of what was being served, or worse yet, didn't eat at all.

A special acknowledgment goes to all the readers of the first edition of the book who gave me feedback. Your support was essential, as were your questions, thoughts, and criticisms. I have no doubt that the feedback you gave was crucial for me to edit and finalize a more interesting book. I must also thank my teachers throughout the times, who gently pushed me to always go slightly beyond my current comfort zone in any project I decided to take on. These include

[Type here]

Marla Sokolowski (my PhD supervisor) and Wanda Viegas (my boss in the genetics department at the University in Lisbon). You inspired and encouraged me to become who I am, and I could have never done this without you. Also, I would have never done this journey if I hadn't taken a one year health coaching course at the Institute for Integrative Nutrition in New York.

To my dear friends and family, the book club girls, my friends in the beach ultimate community, my team, and my science buddies, I cannot express enough gratitude for the fact that you are in my life. There is no way I can ever repay all your support or your concern. Mom, I am fine, ever after eating a load of fat for a month! My health coach, Patricia Oliveira, also deserves special mention. For being patient with me when I was losing it during some of the challenges, for encouraging me when I was feeling weak, and for brain storming as well as supporting me throughout with great recipes, I thank you from the bottom of my heart.

Lastly, and most importantly, a huge amount of gratitude and love goes to my husband and kids, who live with me and put up with me daily. Patrick, Sara and Tomas, I could not have done this without you! As much as I tried not to interfere in your eating choices, I know I did and I thank you for being flexible and taking it in stride. I am also extremely grateful for your constant support, love, and for putting up with my endless discussions of food and food theory. I love you and thank you and can only strive to be my best self because of you.

Introduction

Here we are at the beginning, even though it is the end that we tend to focus on and the process itself that counts.

H. Sofia C. Pereira, 2017

I can't believe that it has been almost one year and a half since I finished my thirty-day food challenges project and published the first edition of this book. Thinking back, I am ever aware that the experience of doing twelve consecutive challenges was quite the trip… and that it forever changed me. Also, the task of completing a self-edited and self-published book was huge!

Digging into my mental archives, I realize that the concept of writing a novel has crossed my mind many times throughout the years. In fact, I believe that a fantastic bestseller could have materialized from the all-too-frequent head scratching personal and family situations that I have experienced over the last decade. But that would be too personal, and I don't like the idea of sharing other people's intimate lives in a public forum. Funny that in the end my first book turned out to be a personal journey through food and drink challenges, which can get fairly intimate… but these are my intimacies to share.

If we consider that food is the prime material

used to construct our physical selves, eating is likely the most intimate thing that we will ever do in our lives. Not only does the food we eat provide the building blocks for our bodies and brains, eating is one of the few things that we do daily and many times a day from the day we are born to the day we die, together with sleeping and going to the bathroom. Since it was precisely my experiments with food challenges that motivated me to write down my thoughts, plans, and scientific research results, this is a book about my intimate food behaviors. Also, considering that the main body of the book is a dairy, I am aware of how personal it can be.

Written as a personal log, I know that this book may seem to be a bit too much about me. Hopefully, that will not be the case as you read and get inspired to explore your own food journey. I really hope that you can connect with some of the things you read and turn them into part of your reality. My hope is that what you read inspires you to make connections to your own experiences, and then create your own path. In the perfect world, you will think about what you read and apply it or use it in a positive way in your life.

In truth, what I would really like is for you to enjoy reading the entire book, from the beginning to the end. As a scientist, I couldn't help delving into the literature on nutrition theory. If you find that some of the content gets too much into scientific details for your liking, I apologize and strongly suggest you just skip those sections. I have tried to write in such a way that it is always worth continuing to read, even after having skipped a part that you are not interested in.

Now, let me tell you how this book came to be. What started this whole thing was my desire to help a client with chronic digestion issues who wanted to try to take gluten out of her diet. I thought it would help me help her if I also removed gluten from my own diet. After a few gluten free weeks, I found that the lessons from the limitation were very, which pushed me to expand the time and eventually the number of limitations, or challenges. In the end, this adventure turned out to be a twelve month stint of consecutive thirty-day challenges involving various food (and beverage) limitations. At this point I am re-editing the first edition of this book, with the namesake of the original file saved in my computer: "the food anthropologist". The title remains, as it is the best way to describe a one year long experiment through twelve food regimes which are currently followed by many around the world.

The experimental period was from May 2016 to May 2017, and the time length of each of the twelve challenges was always twenty-nine or thirty days. Since I decided to use the day of the month rather than to actually count out thirty days for each challenge, the first nine experiments started on the fifth of each month and ended on the third of the following month, with the fourth being a much cherished day off without food limits. The tenth challenge, the paleolithic diet, happened to be in February, which only had twenty-eight days in 2017. To ensure consistency, this challenge was therefore prolonged until the fifth of March, which therefore shifted the last two challenges to initiate on the seventh of their respective months.

There was no specific logic regarding the order in which the diets were done, except for the fact that the initial challenge was inspired directly by a client and the second by an upcoming trip to the United Kingdom. Mostly, the choice of what diet to do next was based on how I felt the last week of the ongoing challenge. Looking in retrospect now, I would risk saying that I gained momentum as the year went on. I will discuss this in further detail throughout the book.

You will notice that even thought this is a book about food, there are no food pictures. There is a reason for that. This is not meant to be a recipe book or even a food book. I actually consider it to be more similar to a travel log. Keep in mind, I do love to cook and have learnt to photograph food, so I frequently posted pictures of the foods cooked and eaten throughout the year. You will easily find these on my Instagram (@sofia.c.pereira/), tagged with #30daychallenge and then with further hashtags with the specific challenge of the month. I mostly cook without recipes, but rather through inspiration from the cooking and recipes of others, which I adapt to my tastes as well as to the ingredients currently in the house. So, if you see something you would like to eat and the recipe is not posted, send me an e-mail and I will be happy to help you out.

For clarity, the motivation of for this 12-month experiment was not to lose weight or to change my body shape. However, I did collect numbers on some metrics after each challenge, such as waist perimeter and weight. Also, compelled by many people annoying me about the effects of some of the regimes on my health, I did blood analysis after the ketogenic month and at the end of all the challenges. This data is sprinkled throughout specific sections of the book as well as demonstrated in a summarized form at the end of the book.

There is one thing that I must make very clear. This work is not intended to be a scientific publication or a therapeutic tool. Rather, it is a qualitative analysis of twelve food experiments, or thirty-day challenges, done consecutively over a one year period. Whatever opinions I have are my personal views and obviously influenced by my subjective feelings, and by no means meant to be objective "absolute truths". What about the specifics of each food and drink challenge? How deep did I delve into each experience?

The answer to those questions is paramount to the existence of this book. I did not just impose specific eating limitations on myself for a month and then move on to the next one. As a scientist and a health coach, I thrive on digging into the literature (scientific publications) to get insight into the biological effects of diets and lifestyles. Of course, this was even more so during the experimental year, where my interest was highly augmented by personally experiencing symptoms or effects of specific diets.

Being a complete fan of knowledge as well as on feedback from my geeky friends who read the original book, I have slightly expanded the scientific component in this edition. Regarding the science in this book, I think it is important to make clear that my opinions are exactly that, opinions. That said, they are informed opinions and are supported by solid literature as listed in the reference list of each chapter. Also, please note that scientific knowledge is continuously growing and theories are constantly adjusting to newly acquired data. Therefore, relevant scientific conclusions from works that have been published in the last year and a half have been included in this revised version.

The format of the book is simple and hopefully easy to read. Each experiment or thirty-day challenge is presented as a separate chapter and contains random entries within the thirty-day period. At the end of each section, there is a short paragraph with a conclusion as well as a list of pros and cons that I felt during that challenge. This part of the book has been minimally edited since the initial log document, much of it written long before the concept of a book materialized.

To give insight into the long-term influence of each specific limitation, I have also added an "in retrospect" paragraph or two at the end of each chapter, which was written in the few months following the completion of all twelve monthly challenges. These in retrospect sections, which are presented in italics, are meant to discuss the impact of specific limitations as well as how they fit into the context of the whole. Also, I have asked my husband and kids a few questions about how these twelve months affected them and what they thought about it. Their wonderful words can be found in the final section, entitled "afterthoughts", which wraps up my experiments and hopefully ties up all loose ends.

Before we go on, let us focus on the most important part of this whole project, the reader... which is you. I really hope you connect with the book and that you look forward to reading it every time you pick it up. As I mentioned before, I have written and published a lot of science in scientific journals, and I have never worried about whether the reader was enjoying my writing. Now I worry. I want you to enjoy it and to be partially sad that it is over when you get to the end and read the final word. Not only do I hope you have fun reading this, I also hope that the content of the book is informative, and that the science is interesting enough for you to learn something.

Perhaps you have thought about trying a new diet. If that is the case, I think you may find the daily log of your diet choice interesting and perhaps helpful. Over the experimental year, I became ever aware of the lack of general knowledge of food intolerances, limitations or eating styles. As I see it, food culture is not a bad thing to be informed about. I would love if my experiences inspire you to try to explore your own food self. No matter what your background or profession, I believe that trying new healthy foods and going beyond your current eating habits only brings advantages.

There is little doubt that variety is important when it comes to what we eat. This is obvious by just thinking of a key phrase commonly used to promote healthy eating, "eat a rainbow every day". And this, of course, does not mean eating a handful of colorful candy daily. Rather, the rainbow reference means eating a wide variety of wholesome fresh foods, and mostly refers to the enormous diversity of colors in edible plants.

A daily menu with a variety of plant foods provides us with all kinds of nutrients in their natural form, which builds us as well as feeds the symbiotic organisms that inhabit our gut. This incredibly complex population of bacteria and other living things (virus, fungus and archaea bacteria) play an extremely relevant role on our physical and mental health. In the scientific literature, these organisms are referred to as the microbiota, and the bacteria as the microbiome.

Many studies have shown that the population of microorganisms in our guts is highly adaptable and responsive to what we eat, and that there are alterations in specific species in the guts of people with numerous diseases or pathologies. According to the latest research, the human gut microbiota consists of trillions of microbial cells and thousands of bacterial species. Thus far, it is not easy to identify what a "healthy" microbiota is, due to the large amount of variability between individuals as well as the fact that their proportions can quickly change.

In general, a gut (poop) rich in micro-organisms and high species variability are both indicators of health. This is obvious by the inverse association between these parameters with chronic disease and metabolic dysfunction. As we get a better understanding into the lifecycles of our symbiotic gut co-habitants, it is becoming clear that they form a functional bio-community. From a practical perspective, it is good for us to eat whole foods that are rich in fiber, as it is precisely the fiber that we cannot digest that feeds them and allows them to help our bodies (including our brains) stay healthy.

Enough of the health lesson, let us talk about food. Trying new foods and recipes is not always easy, but it can be great fun if taken in stride. Also, as we expand our food repertoire and cooking comfort zone, successes such as great "quickly invented" recipes with what is available in the cupboard and fridge become more frequent. Needless to say, great meals give us great pleasure. Considering that we eat every day many times a day, it is worth the investment to explore with foods and enjoy eating.

Of course, we must keep in mind the timing of when we try something completely new... it is never a good idea to wear brand new shoes for a ten-kilometer marathon. New foods should be introduced gradually, so we get a chance to feel how our bodies react. For example, although we may not deal well if we eat a bowl of whole grains just before we go for an intense workout, we could possibly feel great if we ate the same bowl and then went for a long slow hike. When it comes to our eating choices, we must be smart... but should not forget that we tend to put our heads in front of our bodies and not the other way around. Yes, we should use our intelligent brains, but always listening to our bodies and follow instincts.

I really hope you enjoy reading my log through monthly regimes and that it motivates you to do your own food experiments. There is no doubt that self-imposed experiments and can be highly positive on a personal level, regardless of who you are or what you do. If you are a health professional or are close to someone with a food intolerance, these kinds of initiatives are a great way to walk the talk. Living through something ourselves allows us to feel what it is like to eat a certain way, which helps us better support others that are undergoing the same or similar regimes. The personal investment motivates greater involvement and deeper desire to study further, which in turn allows us to better support our clients, family members, or friends that follow a food regime.

In conclusion, I hope my experiences provide insight into following a specific diet and inspire you to widen your food repertoire. Not only is learning about lifestyles of philosophies around diet interesting from a cultural point of view, food awareness is health promoting. Excluding the "no coffee" and "no alcohol" challenges which were liquid challenges and stand by themselves, most of the food challenges, , resulted in increased knowledge and awareness of the consumption of processed foods. Refined and processed foods are not only bad for us, they are also the hardest on our ecosystem.

While reading, I seriously hope you will consider taking a challenge. In the end, you may be amazed by the huge amount of self-discipline which is enabled.

This translates into self-empowerment, and often gives us the push to continue to explore our healthy selves.

And now, here's is my log of a highly interesting year. I hope you enjoy it!

Chapter 1 – gluten free

This challenge was inspired by a client with chronic stomach and intestinal issues. After decades of going for medical exams and talking to doctors with no avail, and having heard of the incredible damage that gluten can do to the intestinal wall, my client decided to take gluten out of her own diet. After our conversation, I decided to not eat any foods with gluten for two weeks, so I could better support my client.

Considering the huge amount of attention and bad press that gluten is getting, there is a lot of miss information out there. To start, let us discuss what gluten is, and then what we know about its effect on health.

To put it simply, gluten is a protein complex (proteins are a type of biological molecule), of which gliadin and glutenin are the main components. It is found in the endosperm of seeds from wheat and its relatives, including rye, barley and spelt, and is often referred to as the storage protein in grains. It's gluey consistency is what gives the elasticity to wheat flour products, such as pasta and bread dough.

Over the last decade, the frequency of diagnoses for gluten-related disorders is rising, evidenced by the increasing numbers of people trying a gluten-free diet for a variety of signs and symptoms. However, there are different types of gluten intolerance with varying degrees of severity. Celiac disease is a genetic disorder in which the individual must not eat gluten. On the other hand, nonceliac gluten sensitivity is diagnosed in those who do not have celiac disease or wheat allergy but who have symptoms related to eating gluten, which disappear once gluten is removed from the diet. Importantly, we do not currently know the prevalence of celiac disease or of nonceliac gluten sensitivity.

A recent review published in JAMA provides insight into the difficulty distinguishing between celiac disease and nonceliac gluten sensitivity (Leonardo et al 2017). Celiac disease is a genetic disorder in which a gluten induced immune mediated condition results in an inflammatory process that attacks the inner intestinal wall (mucosa). Regarding cure, people with celiac disease must be helped to maintain a strict gluten free diet and checked for possible nutrient deficiencies. As a systemic disease, regular checkups are important for celiac disease symptom prevention and treatment.

Regarding non-celiac gluten sensitivity, I think the rise in gluten related symptoms is in great part due to how we process wheat and how we utilize it for processed foods. When taken from the plant, the gluten containing grains have a seed coat and a bunch of other components such as the embryo of the plant. These are stripped away and discarded to make refined flour, which is rich in simple carbohydrates (starch). Digestion of this refined flour is completely different from digestion of the entire seed, as the starch is almost completely devoid of fiber. It is exactly the fiber in the rest of the seed (which has been stripped away) that slows down digestion and ensures that the microbiota in the gut get some nutrition as well. This, not to mention the bleaching and other treatments often done to refined flours.

Let me change channels now and go back to discussing wheat. Wheat, most commonly ground into flour, is used for pasta, bread, dumplings, and other foods. That is the other problem with wheat, we eat a lot of it! As a scientist in an Agronomical Institute, I witnessed many talks about wheat, and how it was going to save our growing population from hunger. Unfortunately, in my opinion, the agro-industry has focused on producing huge amounts of wheat with extreme measures, with various negative effects on the planet as well as on the quality of the grain.

The reality is that gluten has gotten a load of bad press and that there are many people who do not eat gluten containing foods. There are also many others who avoid eating gluten, or do it consciously. On the other hand, wheat agriculture covers more of our planet than any other crop. We eat a lot of wheat flour!

The day before

Three days ago, a client of mine mentioned that she was interested in trying to cut gluten from her diet to see if it helped resolve her chronic stomach issues. After our talk, and thinking about the much-publicized gluten sensitivities and intolerances, I started to become interested in how I could best support my client through this change in eating. Looking at my own food choices, I concluded that I eat way too much foods made with wheat flour, especially bread.

Whether because it's the easy choice or because I really do like it, a quick look-into my daily food intake made me realize that I am grabbing for bread at least three times a day. Sometimes it is just a chunk ripped off the loaf that is sitting in the bag on the counter, other times I make myself a sandwich or use bread as an accompaniment in a meal. Let me be clear, it's not that I have anything against bread… nor do I have any gluten sensitivity that I am aware of. I do, however, have something against lack of variety when it comes to my food choices.

Also, maybe cutting out bread for a while will help me lose a couple of kilograms that seem to be very attached to my waistline for the last decade. Taken together, these seem like a good reason to see what happens if I completely cut out gluten from my diet for two weeks.

Day 1

I did not realize that gluten, an integral component of wheat and it's evolutionary relatives such as barley and rye, is everywhere! Today, I became acutely aware that this is not going to be easy, especially for an assumed flexitarian (which, by the way, simply means someone with no food restrictions).

Day 2

Although I am already missing fluffy, elastic wheat bread, I am starting to enjoy the challenge. My stomach feels a bit different… similar to that feeling you get on an empty stomach. Funny, I find myself to always be slightly hungry, even after a good meal.

Day 4

Or is it? Last night, which was day three, I went to meet a friend in downtown Lisbon. After attending a lecture on male/female energy at the Instituto Macrobiótico de Portugal (Portuguese Macrobiotic Institute), we went for dinner at an Asian fusion noodle house. I ordered a noodle dish described on the menu as being prepared with buckwheat pasta, which does not contain gluten. When dinner arrived, I found the noodles themselves to be surprisingly flexible and lacking the characteristic nutty buckwheat taste. I have to admit though, it was ten o'clock at night and I was starved, and ended up devouring the whole thing trying hard not to eat too fast.

Afterwards, I asked the waitress how the noodles were made and quickly realized by the puzzled look on her face that she had no clue what I was asking. The conversation went something like this:

I asked, "Could you please tell me what the pasta in my soup was made from?"

And she responded, looking smug, "Wheat, and it's homemade."

Then I said, "But it says on the menu that it was made from buckwheat, which is very different from wheat and has no gluten."

To which she retorted "I only said it was made from wheat flour, I did not say it had gluten."

I felt my face getting hot while rationalizing with myself that this interaction was quickly turning into a conversation not worth exploring. In the end, I left the restaurant irritated and feeling unresolved on whether I had eaten gluten or not. On the way home, I thought about how difficult it must be to have serious issues with gluten, like for example to have gluten sensitivity or intolerance, as is the case for those with celiac disease. After getting home and about one hour after eating, I had loads of gases and felt bloated, but was it the gluten or some of the other salts and additives they tend to put in Asian food? I will never know but I did learn a big lesson, that if I am really going to do a serious experiment and cut out gluten completely, I must be more careful about what I put in my mouth. Regardless of whether my noodles were gluten free or not, today I'm craving bread and intend to walk to the health food store later to buy some gluten free flour variety or bread.

Day 8

I lasted one week, woohoo! Proud to be here!

This is not an easy experiment for a bread fanatic, although I must admit it is getting easier. As I wrote in my last entry, which was on a Friday, I did go to the health food store to shop for gluten free bread, and bought a loaf made with corn flour. Unfortunately, it looked absolutely disgusting and very similar to that horrible packaged white loaf breads that I haven't eaten since high school over thirty years back.

As bad as it was, I toasted it and ate it accompanied by tea, and I have been missing bread so much that I enjoyed it. However, while eating my toast, I realized I needed to find an alternative for my bread cravings... thank goodness that when it comes to what we put in our mouths, there are always alternatives!

And so began my search and find of alternative bread recipes. Over the weekend, which corresponded to gluten free days five and six, I made all kinds of wholesome and yummy gluten free breads and other goodies. For baking, I used homemade whole rice and/or chickpea flour. What a pleasure to bake and to eat. The house smelt wonderful, and the kids loved everything I made!

Saturday morning started off with chickpea and rice flour pancakes and then a trip to the health food store to buy psyllium husks for a rice flour/psyllium husk/milk bread recipe. Sunday morning, I baked a fresh loaf. My health coach's recipe made the best bread! Loved it then and am still enjoying it two days later. Thank-you Patricia!

Besides all the cooking and baking, do I feel different after one gluten free week? I think so. I feel like I have less of a belly and am "thinning out". This is probably because I tended to eat a fair bit of bread and am therefore just eating less. I am also enjoying the experience from an anthropological point of view – both scientifically and behaviorally.

Removing gluten from my diet has affected the options and lack of them when eating out; what to shop for and to cook; what pasta alternatives are there that serve as easy family dinner options, etc. At least one more week and then we'll see what I do. Maybe I will weigh myself tomorrow (which I haven't yet) so I can track any changes in weight. If I was asked right now whether I would repeat the experiment, my answer would be a resounding YES!

Day 9

I am hungry and in dire desire of some fluffy, flexible, crusty, chewy and wonderful smelling wheat bread from my favorite bakery next door, called *A Merenda*! Amazing how up and down this experiment has been... some days I think that this is exactly what I need and other days, like today - which is rainy and cold for Portuguese standards in May, I feel that I am insane to put myself through this torture. I still haven't weighed myself, so maybe that is the answer. Since I quit smoking almost two and a half years ago, and decided not to weigh myself for at least one year so as not to despair, I tend to forget to step on the balance and leave those metrics up to my less than yearly visits to the doctor. I guess now is the time, so I'm off to do that and then to exercise. Hopefully that will get my mind off gluten rich bread and pasta!

Back from doing a workout and then stepping on the balance, and the results were 61 kg in track pants and long sleeve t-shirt just after lunch. Although I am committed to re-weighing myself tomorrow morning before breakfast, this has been my normal weight for the last few years, and I would like to reduce it by a few kilograms.

Day 10

My morning weight in undies was 60.3 kg. Today I am making another gluten free bread loaf to take to my aunt who just got out of the hospital for knee surgery.

Day 13

One more gluten free weekend! I am extremely proud

to have gotten through this last weekend, I have to admit... especially considering that we had a birthday dinner party with lots of very appetizing and undoubtedly delicious wheat based foods.

Now I know why people that don't eat gluten are generally thinner. It is much more difficult to over eat without eating bread or cracker type appetizers, and with pasta main dishes and cakes for desert being off limits. I did make a great chickpea bread yesterday, so one good thing is that I now feel completely comfortable whipping up my own flour in the food processor by using seeds, whole grain rice, and various nuts or legumes and then using it to bake bread.

Day 14

Today is the final day of the two-week long gluten free experiment and I seriously screwed up, I drank beers! Here goes what happened, full disclosure. A girlfriend of mine is going through a tough break up, and dropped by for support as well as to vent. I met her at the train station and then we walked to the beach, where we ended up sitting at a bar and drinking beers! I completely forgot about my gluten free challenge, and only when happily downing my third small draft beer did I realize what I was doing. Within one hour, I felt like I swallowed an entire cow, a feeling that remained for the rest of the day. I am not sure if it was the gluten or the fact that I haven't touched beer in two weeks. I do feel bad about it, but decided to chalk it up to experience... like the coaching specialists say "look at your failures with curiosity".

On another note, I have decided to continue with this experiment for a while longer.

Day 20

Almost three weeks into this challenge and I am doing well and getting creative with gluten free cooking. I decided to extend the gluten free experiment for a full month. I did weigh in yesterday at minus 300 g and think I may be a bit thinner. The question remains whether it is it the gluten, or simply the fact that I am so limited in what I can eat. I don't know, but we will see what happens after the month. Also, I decided to do more food experiments as I find them really enriching from an anthropological point of view.

Speaking of challenges, I think I have already decided what the next experiment will be. Considering that I will be travelling a lot, and that I am a coffee addict, it seems to be a great time to go without coffee for one month. As is always the case with our conscious decisions, there are many more reasons why this will come in handy…

Day 24

Today, I feel like I have had enough of the gluten free, although I will hang in there for one more week. I so look forward to having some yum wheat bread in the morning and to eat a great pasta dish. To be honest, I think these desires mostly arise from being sick of having culinary limitations and not being able to eat the things I enjoy. Like most people, I do not like to be told what to do. As I age, I notice that I am becoming increasingly anarchic and less and less into fitting into someone else's idea of what should be. Ok, enough philosophizing… got to hang in there one more week!

Day 28

Counting down the days until there are no restrictions on what I eat. It's not the gluten free per se, I actually enjoy a lot of gluten free foods. It is just that I am sick of not being able to eat everything. On the other hand, I weighed myself today and I am down another 100 g. I also measured my waist circumference and it has reduced by 2 cm compared to the first day I weighed myself. I guess taking out gluten is doing something positive in that regard. In the end, I think this challenge has had many positive effects, such as the fact that I have learnt how to make different flours and breads without using the bread machine. Will it have long-term effects on my eating habits? Probably.

Day 30

Last gluten free day and I can't wait until it's over! It seems that I have reached the point that I am constantly feeling irritated by the limitation. I can see the positive side of the experience, but I am getting cravings for sugary stuff and believe that these are related to the fact that I can't have a slice of bread or a bowl of pasta. This week, I bought "semi unhealthy white flour" bagels, cream cheese and smoked salmon to enjoy on my day off.

I am really looking forward to digging my teeth into the gluten rich wheat flour bagels for breakfast tomorrow, which I will accompany with a large cup of piping hot Dutch-style coffee with milk, the last coffee breakfast for a while…

Conclusion

In the end, I am very glad that I did a gluten free month. From an experimental point of view, these 30 days were enriching in many ways. First of all, they definitely changed my all too frequent habit of eating bread. Also, going gluten free pushed me to learn how to make breads and bake with different flours, such as chickpea, almond, oat and rice.

As a result of this experiment, eating wheat flour bread stopped being part of my daily routine, which means that I will most likely eat less gluten in the future. The realization that gluten (from wheat or other gluten containing cereals such as spelt, barley, and rye) was everywhere was also an eye opener. It makes me question if we simply eat too much of it and therefore have become partially intolerant.

We will see how my future relationship with this highly mediatized complex molecule present in wheats and their ancestors goes. For now and to wrap up this month, here are the positives and negatives as I see them.

Positives

- Weaned off the frequent daily (2-3 times a day, on average) bread meals or snacks.
- Explored with making different flours and baking various breads.

- Could not eat sugary cakes or baked goods in bakeries or when out for dinner.
- Lost 1 kg in 1 month, likely due to not being able to eat a lot of the options available away from home.
- Lost 2 cm waist circumference.
- Had regular bowel and intestinal movements.
- Learnt about Psyllium husks.

Negatives
- Hate having food limitations.
- Parties and social gatherings were difficult.
- Felt gassy, especially in the first two weeks and probably due to adjustments to diet changes.
- Felt lack of energy, also especially the first two weeks and likely for the same reasons as above.
- Could not drink beer (except for screw up on day 14).
- Kids and husband complained that they miss pasta at mealtimes.
- Felt constantly hungry.

My day off

Oh yay-woop-yay, no food limits! I enjoyed a bagel with cream cheese and smoked salmon this morning for breakfast, accompanied by a large cup of Dutch style coffee with milk. It tasted great! So far, no symptoms from having consumed wheat for the first time in a long time. We'll see how it goes, but I right now I am seriously looking forward to an ice-cold beer later on tonight!

In retrospect

More than an entire year has gone by since I did this challenge, and I am in awe reading about how difficult it was for me to go gluten-free for a month. Did it change how I eat? Yes, it definitely has. I currently don't eat as much bread or pasta as I used to. In fact, my whole family eats less pasta, and what used to be a once a week dinner choice for us is currently probably closer to being a once a month option or less. But considering that many challenges were done after the gluten free month, I am finding it hard to pinpoint how this specific month changed my or our eating habits.

In retrospect, I enjoyed the realization that the decision to go on with consecutive food experiments only happened sometime halfway into this particular challenge, and that there were no intentions to do them for a full year. Also, it is very cool to see that it was the only food experiment in which I cheated, and unconsciously or not, ate gluten twice throughout the month. On one hand, it shows that a it is what is part of our routines that really counts, and two isolated (involuntary) cheats do not take away from the validity of the year.

Like I often tell my clients, screw ups are inevitable, it is how long it takes us to recover from them that counts. So, in the end, I am happy that the damage was contained into two isolated cheats rather than becoming an excuse to give up.

Gluten-free revisited – November 2018

We have been eating and cultivating wheat and its

relatives for approximately 8000 years, and wheat flour is considered a "staple food" for many. On a global level, I think we eat too much refined flour, which unfortunately is often paired with sugars and unhealthy fats (in prepackaged cakes, cookies, pastries, and cereal bars). When it comes to digestion, refined flour based foods are rich in easily absorbed carbs. Although this can be very useful in sports, refined flour has low nutritional value and high inflammatory potential once it makes up a large part of the daily diet.

There is no doubt that gluten has received a lot of bad press lately. Just today, I had a very difficult time finding Seitan on the google, after having forgotten the name of a food consisting of gluten and water. This protein rich food, which is basically wheat flour washed away of starch, was often used as a protein choice for vegan meals. I have cooked it a few times, and have also enjoyed it out in vegetarian restaurants. Although it is a processed food, Seitan fills me up like a meal with animal protein. From a nutritional point of view, it would be interesting to see if the sensitivity to gluten is different if it is not ingested with starch.

The reality is that we need to eat a variety of plant foods because we need their fiber to keep our intestinal tracts and guts healthy. Ideally, a rainbow of plants provide different plant phytochemicals, nutrients, and even different fibers. Keep in mind that whenever we eat too much of one thing, we don't have space for other things. Rather than cutting out foods and ingredients, introducing healthy options often crowds out less healthy foods, or foods that we eat too much of. Exploring the wonderful world of whole grains, for example, is a much healthier way to eat cereals, and there are plenty gluten free options. As always, variety is key!

References

Leonard MM, Sapone A, Catassi C, Fasano A. 2017. Celiac Disease and Nonceliac Gluten Sensitivity: A Review. JAMA. 2017. Vol 318(7), pp. 647

Chapter 2 – coffee free

My second experiment is to go without coffee for a month. The reason I chose this challenge is somewhat similar to the reason for going gluten free, I know that I drink way too much coffee. Especially after having quit smoking two and a half years ago, I can easily drink three expressos in a day, sometimes straight up and sometimes with a drop of milk or milk foam. Thank goodness I don't like sugar in my coffee.

Regarding my coffee addiction, I would like you to keep in mind that drinking multiple coffees a day is quite a common practice in Portugal, where expressos often start the day and cap off every meal. Anyway, I am aware of the effects of coffee on me and that it has become an all too frequent habit. Taken together with the fact that I will be travelling to the land of tea (UK) for the next month to work at the world championships of grass ultimate, marks now as the perfect time to go without my liquid gold for 30 days.

Day 1

The first thing I did this morning was to go to my neighborhood café *A Merenda*, stand at the counter, and wait until they served me my perfect foamy expresso. As I was standing there, it sunk in… no coffee for this chick! Oh boy! I was grateful that the gluten free stint was done and bought bread, and then went home feeling like something was missing. The whole day I had a slight headache and felt sleepy. We will see if I can go a whole month without my beloved "cafézinho".

The Portuguese, like me, characteristically love their coffee. It is part of our culture. This is obvious by the many ways to say coffee in Portugal. It's actually interesting that many of them don't even have the word coffee in them, such as "bica", which is the typical way to ask for an expresso in the Lisbon area, or "cimbalino" (the name of a classical expresso machine) often used in Porto.

There is also "galão" (coffee with milk served in a tall glass), "meia de leite" (half coffee and half milk served in a shallow mug), "pingado" (the word means with a drop and is used to order an expresso with a touch of milk or some strong alcoholic beverage, for example Portuguese moonshine) and at least five more that I can think of (garoto, escaldado, curto, cheio, carioca). Coffee is a much-loved bean in my small corner of the world.

Day 2
Still have a headache, still want a coffee, still not sure if I can do this.

Day 3
No headache today, but still feeling a bit fuzzy and craving coffee. I'm getting cravings for sweets and am slightly afraid that I will compensate my lack of coffee with junk food. Oh, I must hold out and be strong.

Day 8

Finally, after a full week of struggling with all-over sluggishness, a clear mind and no more headache. I am glad to know that I can read, concentrate, assimilate, connect, create, think, focus and function without coffee! Thank goodness, as I do have some writing to do and I just hate "fuzzy head writing". Today is a good day, and I am feeling strong and healthy and am still not eating much gluten - maximum one serving a day. And hopefully starting today, feeling energetic again!

Day 12

Patrick and I are off to London to go to the World Ultimate and Guts Championships (WUGC2016) and I hope it will not be too difficult not to drink coffee. I feel like I have been eating a little too many sweets for my liking in the last few days, and it worries me to think how I will compensate for the lack of coffee the following three weeks, which will be crazy.

First, we are going to London for a few weeks to work with ERIC, which stands for Early Recognition is Critical, a non-for-profit organization that teaches the sport of ultimate frisbee as a vehicle for educating youth about cancer symptom awareness and to speak up when they feel something is wrong. I am really looking forward to that, and think it is an important cause.

Right after London, we are coming back into Lisbon and immediately packing off to Meco to play and party at the 20th edition of the Bar do Peixe Beach Ultimate Frisbee tournament (BDP) for four days. With eleven games on soft beach and lots of late nights and parties over the four days, BDP is an endurance test or physical challenge in itself.

Looking at things from a positive perspective, at least I won't be overdoing it on coffee. Although truth be told, I expect to be eating and drinking a fair bit of non-health promoting stuff for the next three weeks.

Day 18

It has been insanely busy in London at the WUGC2016. Our ERIC booth is in the same tent as the bar, and since we often don't have a chance to leave the booth and go get food, we end up feeding mostly on beer during the day. If I could drink coffee, I would probably be overdoing it on that as well.

Every day, I am amazed at how difficult it is not to cheat... especially at breakfast and while working at the booth where fresh coffee smell wafts in from the coffee stand nearby. I am often close to cheating, especially because I had forgotten how much I actually like crappy coffee with milk and sugar. In fact, back in my PhD days in Toronto, I did some of my best genetics work (complex classical genetics crosses in Drosophila) with a huge cup of Tim Horton's coffee with double cream.

But I haven't cheated, and thanks to English breakfast tea, have managed ok.

Day 30

Still coffee free - and it has been really tough! This also means that I survived the first Bar do Peixe (BDP) without my critical and much needed morning coffee (note that morning at BDP means 2 pm after a night of going to bed when the sun is already up) and after dinner expressos!

Oh, I am just now having a brain fart... the lack of coffee may explain why I was so pooped and ended up struggling to keep my eyes open at the two of the four parties of the tournament. That makes me happy, as I prefer that my tiredness be explained by lack of coffee than by the thought that I am just getting old and therefore not able to enjoy myself at late parties. Well, it's done and I did it - one more challenge met! I am proud to have succeeded and looking forward to doing more.

Conclusion

Not drinking coffee for a month was much more difficult than I thought and I am very happy to have gotten through it. At the beginning of the 30 days, I was surprised at how strong the physical symptoms of coffee withdrawal were. Especially the first week, when I felt stupid, fuzzy headed, tired and not functional. Thank goodness that the initial horrible phase was quick to pass, although it did make me realize how off quilter and addicted my body was.

Positives
   - Weaned off an addiction.
   - Managed to do what I said I would even thought it was hard, which is great for my ego.
   - Will not drink 3-4 coffees a day anymore (I hope).

- Eventually got a clear functional mind back without the coffee (took one week).

Negatives
  - I do not like limits!
  - Had many sugar cravings.
  - Found that not being able to use coffee as a recreational wake up drug after dinner resulted in party nights being less fun because I was sleepier.
  - Weighed in at 61.4 Kg, which means i gained approximately 2 kg this month. However, this was more likely due to the crappy eating and drinking associated with travel than to the no coffee challenge itself.

My day off

This morning started with one of my all-time favorite breakfasts, a piping hot and strong "galão", which is similar to a latte and served in a tall glass, accompanied by toasted Portuguese rustic bread with butter! I am very happy to be finished with this experiment, but am also happy to have put a stop to my coffee addiction.

Considering that the gluten free experiment did result in me eating much less bread, my target from now on is to reduce my coffee intake. I hope to drink a maximum of two coffees a day, and keep it to one except on special days.

And now on to month three! I am still undecided what my next challenge will be, which starts tomorrow!

In retrospect

I can only smile as I write this immediately after I come back from my second expresso of the day. One year later, and I am likely exactly where I was before I did this challenge as far as my coffee consumption is concerned. I probably drink two to three coffees a day, which means that my resolution to keep it to one or two a day did not hold out.

I am aware of my "coffee-holic" tendencies, and often stop myself from walking to my friendly corner café and ordering a "cafézinho" every time I feel like it. Does my coffee consumption worry me? No, not at all. I feel great and healthy and would likely drink way less coffee if lived in a place that the coffee wasn't so good and cheap (I pay 65 cents per expresso at my favorite café, Merenda).

My relationship with coffee and current coffee consumption are completely contrary to the long-term effects of "weaning off an addiction" from bread that I felt and still feel after the first gluten free challenge. Going without gluten for a month has made an impact on me to this day, I eat significantly less wheat flour than I used to.

No coffee revisited – November 2018

I am still in love with coffee. There is nothing better than a cup of coffee and a book in bed on weekend mornings, and I cherish my comings and goings to A Merenda (the local café/bakery) for coffee with Patrick. Besides all the wonderful anti-oxidants that coffee has, along with tea and red wine, the health benefits of coffee for me include the pleasure that I gain from it... and likely always will.

Chapter 3 – ovo-lacto vegetarian

After much pondering over the last 24 hours about what challenge to do next, I have decided that my third food experiment is to not eat meat or fish for the next month. As the name "ovo-lacto vegetarian" implies, I am permitted to eat eggs and dairy.

Happily, I have company for this challenge. As soon as I announced the decision to not eat animal flesh, my daughter Sara told me she is going to join me. Let's see how this goes, but somehow I think it will be the easiest challenge so far.

Day 2

Two days into fleshless food and nothing feels different or out of the normal. This is likely due to this eating style being very similar to how I normally eat, which typically includes various dairy products, eggs and a lot of plant based foods.

This evening should be interesting. We are going downtown into Lisbon to have dinner while watching Portugal play Wales in the EURO semi-final soccer game. Portugal is not the best place for nutritionally challenged people to eat out, and I'm curious if it will be difficult to get a good dinner without meat or fish.

Day 3

I woke up feeling sick today with a summer flu. Considering the physical demands of the last few weeks, including the crazy time in London followed by the four-day tournament and associated parties, I am not surprised. Summer flu, quick to come, quick to go.

Apart from that, I am still smiling about last night. It turned out to be a great night in Lisbon, starting off with dinner in a cool Portuguese restaurant with an old friend from Canada followed by celebrating a victory for Portugal (2-0) against Wales in a large city square (Terreiro do Paço) full of happy Portuguese people and tourists.

Interesting how difficult it was to eat a healthy meal without animal meat. Luckily, the restaurant served "fish from the orchard", a typical Portuguese tempura like dish made with battered and deep fried green beans. Then there was salad and soup, and that was it for dinner options.

Oh, and Sara is already off the diet. She found the restrictions to be too inconvenient with all the summer barbeques. Plus, she felt rude not eating whatever was being served by her friend's parents when at friend's houses for a meal. I understand and know just how she feels, food restrictions can be very anti-social.

Day 7

Today marks the day that I am one week into this challenge and it is getting tougher. The funny thing is that I think my sub-conscious mind is telling me something through my dreams. Yesterday, Patrick and I watched the EURO final against France at a Pizza place (where I dined on a salad and drank cider) and afterwards celebrated Portugal becoming European soccer champions on the streets of downtown Lisbon.

We got home late, happy and tired, so I fell asleep fast and deep. Overnight, I dreamt about eating raw, live, swimming fish.

This morning, the first thing that went through my mind when I woke up was that I wanted to eat any kind of animal. To be honest, I am not particularly enjoying this experiment and actually feel a bit physically and mentally weak after just one week. Amazing, especially considering that I don't eat that much meat normally. I also don't like that the lack of strength and energy just gets worse if I try to forget my food desires by pushing myself physically and working out, like for example this morning when I went running.

One thing is for sure, I am not going to try to go vegan for a full month. In fact, I am right now really looking forward to the paleolithic diet – give me meat!

Day 10

I still have not eaten any animal flesh and am happy to say that my crazy cravings and weird graphic dreams about eating live animals have died down a bit. Something happened this morning that I have never experienced before, I woke up with cramps in the calf muscles of both my legs. I think it is likely to be related to not eating meats, as is the weakness in my muscles that I feel since a week into this challenge, especially if I run up the stairs or push my body to do something physically more strenuous for more than a few minutes.

I am right now slightly worried about a dinner party that we have tonight. Considering that there will be a set menu, I am curious about whether there will be healthy options. Also, will I come across as rude because I don't eat what is offered to me?

Regarding the logistics of what foods to eat, I don't find it too difficult to be an ovo-lacto vegetarian when I eat at home where the possibilities are endless. I normally don't eat much meat anyway, on average red meat about once a week, chicken once or twice a week and ditto for fish. But going to other people's homes for dinner or eating out at restaurants is a whole new ballgame. It can be very unpleasant being horrible guest that snubs her nose at what is offered.

For the sake of transparency, which I ardently believe in, I feel the need to record that I am going to take 360 mg fish oil tabs for Omega-3 fatty acid, in the hope of offsetting the fatigue and muscle tiredness that has set in. Hopefully it will help. I can't believe that there are still twenty days to go. In the end, this is a serious exercise in self-discipline.

Day 14

I survived another weekend without eating flesh, although it was not easy. Once again, my immediate family of four was invited to a family dinner party in a restaurant to celebrate the 18th birthday of my cousin's and close friend's daughter. At the party, most of the healthy options on the pre-chosen menu consisted of some type of sea carcass. As a result, I drank much more that I ate. Although I had a load of fun celebrating the birthday of someone who is dear and close to me and my family, the self-imposed eating limits were not easy, nor was keeping away from some amazing looking and probably very delicious seafood. To add insult to injury, I felt rude politely and sheepishly turning foods away or leaving them on my plate. By the end of the night, and because there was so little that I could eat and gin and tonics don't have animal protein, I ended up drinking way too much.

The second food related difficulty this past weekend was brought on by a beach ultimate league day with four games held in a gorgeous beach 40 km south of Lisbon. Considering that the party was the night before and went until 4 am, I didn't have time to prepare food to take to the beach. Unfortunately, the beach restaurant had a very limited menu of healthy options for my current eating regime – and bread with crappy cheese accompanied by chips did not seem the least bit appetizing compared to their famous squid dishes.

As these time passes, my biggest beef (no pun intended) with food limitations is that they often do not favor the healthy option, especially when away from home. On a more positive note and taking into account how physically weak I have been feeling lately, I was happy to have been able to play decently and to feel physically strong the entire beach ultimate league day.

Which brings me to the third hurdle of the weekend, my after disc meal. Sadly, as if often the case after doing a lot of sports, I craved red meat after a day running around on the beach. Bearing in mind the current limitations, spicy Indian vegetarian food turned out to be a good alternative. So off Patrick and I went to a local Indian restaurant, both starving, and had a "first" when it comes to the definition of hot-spicy food.

We arrived at the restaurant late after the games, around 10:30 pm on a Sunday night, and were the only costumers there. We were both afraid the kitchen would be closed, and were happy to be led to a table with the promise of a late dinner. Since Patrick and I both love hot-spicy Indian food, we asked for a spicy vegetarian dish. However, the wonderful smelling curry they served us was so spicy that, for the first time in our lives, we just could not eat it. Not even with a load of basmati rice. I have since thought of the possibility that the waiters were unhappy to have to serve us so late, and therefore tried to kill us with capsaicin - the active ingredient in spicy food.

Earlier this evening, I used the leftovers of the vegetarian spicy dish that I brought home in a takeaway container, added a an entire can of chickpeas, more vegetables and a can of coconut milk. Although edible and enjoyed by all, we still found the curry to be just slightly too spicy even after such a large dilution. And this for a family that eats a lot of spice.

Day 20

One more week gone by as an ovo-lacto vegetarian and holding onto my willpower not to cheat, even though I am desperately missing eating animal flesh. Truth be told, I feel that the weakness in my body and the overwhelming desire to eat meat or fish is a telltale sign that this regime is lacking in some vitamins and minerals that my body needs. Once again looking towards solutions, I am aware that only now am I starting to know how to eat within this self-imposed limitation.

I had a very good and satisfying vegetarian meal two nights ago at a vegetarian restaurant in Lisbon. After proper appetizers and a main course of mystic kebob with tofu, pineapple and seitan, I actually felt full for hours and went to bed without a hole in my stomach. This experience has made me think that perhaps I have to adjust how I cook and eat as a vegetarian, and am now looking forward to a special dinner at a vegetarian restaurant for my birthday in a couple of days. On the other hand, I am counting down the days to being able to eat some awesome Portuguese grilled fish.

Day 22

Tomorrow is my 51st birthday, holy cow! How did fifty two years go by? Well, I am happy to be where I am and look forward to the possibility of many more healthy spins around the sun. And now onto the topic at hand, food without meats.

Last night while grocery shopping I actually made sure to buy good protein-rich meat alternatives, such as seitan, tofu and quinoa. Today I made a great lunch consisting of oven baked sweet potatoes and grilled seitan accompanied by red pepper/red cabbage coleslaw. Feeling full and happy and ready to watch the second episode of season six of Game of Thrones.

Funny how my mood changes when I am not feeling nutrient-deficient... maybe I am finally getting the hang of this vegetarian thing.

Day 27

Still hanging in there. Also, I am finally finding it easier not to compensate the lack of animal meat by eating too many eggs or too much cheese, yogurt and nuts. On my birthday (July twenty-seventh), Patrick, the two kids and I went to a great vegetarian restaurant in Cascais called House of Wonders. I loved the food and the minty lemonade and will definitely go back there. Maybe with my daughter, who also adores to go out for lunch and share meals with me.

Other than a few specialized vegetarian or vegan restaurants, Portugal is not easy for those who don't eat meat. Which means that although my meal options at home have changed to fit the ovo-lacto vegetarian lifestyle, it is still extremely difficult to find wholesome options in traditional Portuguese restaurants. For example, Patrick and I went to spend a day with friends by the coast in Peniche a couple of days ago, where the fresh fish and seafood is just amazing. At a sea-side restaurant, I had to contend myself with vegetable soup for lunch and a greasy canned mushroom omelet for dinner.

My limited options were not my first choices for sure, especially watching my husband and friends dig into a beautifully prepared dish of fresh scallops. Anyway, this adventure is almost done. For the sake of consistency, today I have decided that the fourth of every month will be my day off and the fifth day of each month the start of a new experiment.

Day 28

Last night after a great game of disc with my daughter's friends, we ended up inviting a few people over, including one of her friends and one of my friends. Since we got home late and very hungry, the dinner menu consisted of readily prepared vegetarian burgers and spinach sticks baked in the oven with homemade mashed potatoes and endive. This was the first time we are eating previously prepared foods in our house in a long time... which brings me to my next challenge, which will start in four days: no processed foods for a month.

Day 30

Final day as an ovo-lacto vegetarian and feeling ready to bite into some animal flesh and move on to the next challenge. Weighed in this morning at 59.9 Kg.

Conclusion

What an experience this month was! Ovo-lacto vegetarian was much tougher than I expected, especially taking into account that this eating style is not so different from my regular one. Perhaps because it is the third month in a row where I impose a food limitations on myself or perhaps because of the longer-term effects of not eating animal flesh, I felt large differences in how I felt physically this month.

I was interested to note that it took at least two weeks for me to sense that I had finally gotten the hang of how to eat this way without overdoing it on things that I already ate, such as milk, eggs, and cheese. This, of course required introducing foods that did not previously belong in my regular diet, such as seitan, tofu, and husks/seeds.

In general and taking into account my current lifestyle, I do not think I would ever chose this type of diet. It limits the choices of what to eat and often forces me to eat the unhealthy option (such as a gin and tonic). I also believe that the lack of nutrients exclusively present in animal flesh, such as creatine and EPA and DHA Omega fats, resulted in my feeling weaker and less energetic.

The biggest positive outcome of this month was the fact that this is the third food experiment that I complete, and after three months I feel a huge gain in self-discipline and self-trust. Can't wait to see how this whole adventure develops.

Positives
- One more time, I managed to do what I promised myself I would do even thought it was not easy.
- Learnt a lot about cooking with legumes and quinoa as well as other vegetarian protein options such as seitan and tofu.
- Learnt what it means to eat this way and therefore will be able to better support my clients who choose this eating style.
- Realized the importance of animal protein in my diet, especially fish.

- Lost 1.5 Kg in one month without going hungry (keeping in mind that I had 1 kg extra at the beginning of the month from the London trip).

Negatives
- Once again, I do not like having food limits and believe they often lead to choices that are not health promoting.
- The limits led to a tendency of overdoing it on starchy or unhealthy sugary foods.
- Felt serious muscle weakness and woke up in the middle of the night with leg cramps, which had never happened to me before except in the late stages of my pregnancies. These effects were mostly felt in the first two weeks.
- Got the flu, which may be completely unrelated.

My day off

Oh what a treat!

I had a fantastic lunch out with my favorite three people (husband and kids, in case you're wondering) at a great seafood place called Eduardinhos, in Carcavelos. Plenty of seafood including octopus salad and fresh oysters... not bad choices for the first flesh I bite into in a month! Feeling great and ready for a new challenge, which starts tomorrow!

In retrospect

The third adventure in this journey was a surprisingly interesting one for me. Regarding the food limitation, I was not expecting it to be so difficult not to eat meat and fish, and was surprised by my instinctual need for animal flesh, including thoughts of eating live fish while swimming in the ocean or biting into live cows. It was so bizarre that the mental images from those memories are still vivid in my mind. For example, while swimming with my son at the beach in front of our house, I would imagine myself diving down to the small fish swimming beneath me, opening my mouth wide, and swallowing live fish... like a whale. These types of "I need flesh!" instincts often brought to mind a friend from graduate school, and how I could finally relate to him. Back then, I used to get shocked when he would tell us that the first thing that went through his mind when looking at a field of grazing cows was, "Dinner!".

Besides the specifics of ovo-lacto vegetarian month, some interesting things also came up while reading over and editing this third chapter. One is that I now realize that the whole year was not pre-planned at all. Which means that after three months of food challenges, I had no clue how or where this journey would end up. This is clear by reading over what I wrote about vegan, namely that I could never do it.

What I like about this lack of pre-planning is that it shows that I must have enjoyed the process to keep doing it, as well as that it was the process itself that pushed things forward. It gives me a huge amount of satisfaction to see in practice what I constantly preach, that the result is part of the process. Speaking of process, sticking with the plan is what allows for results to eventually be measurable. In this case, after a couple of weeks, there started to be notable differences in the types of foods used at home. Things take time, and if we are patient and persistent, change does occur.

For the sake of completion, I must mention that this is one of the few times I got sick and felt weak throughout the food challenges year. Keeping in mind that it may be purely coincidental, I also got quite sick and felt extremely during the vegan month.

Would I do this regime voluntarily? No, I would not. I thought about it while enjoying that wonderful fresh seafood meal with my family on my day off and many times since. I never want to deprive myself of fresh fish, seafood or organic chicken, pork or beef. In my current life, where I live, with my activity level, etcetera, I believe that the best healthy option for me is to be a flexitarian. But I am glad I did it, I learnt a lot and it was undoubtedly an important part of my progress and food learning curve.

Ovo-lacto vegetarian revisited– November 2018

Looking back on this particular month, which at the time was so difficult for me, I realize how much the ovo-lacto vegetarian regime widened the ingredients commonly found in our fridge and pantry as well as the types of meals we feel happy and comfortable cooking and eating. Considering that over two years have passed, I am happy to announce that these changes have undoubtedly enriched my and my family's experiences with food.

Chapter 4 – whole foods

My fourth food experiment is whole foods – which means that I cannot eat any processed foods for one month! The good news is that I can eat anything that has not been altered by human intervention since it was collected, and I can prepare it how I wish! Off limits are pasta, white flour, sugars, refined grains, any processed meats, and so on. I will have to read labels carefully. What I can eat includes natural milk, yogurt, and other dairy products, eggs, meats, fruits, vegies, and all other natural whole foods. Regarding alcohol, only naturally fermented alcoholic drinks without additives such as organic wine and beer are allowed.

I am looking forward to this one, and since I can eat any type of food, actually believe that will be the easiest challenge to do so far. In fact, my prediction is that although this will be the least difficult challenge, it will be the one with the most impact on my body and how I feel, for the better of course. Today I weigh in at 59.9 kg and have a circumference around my belly button of 87 cm. I am curious to see how eating whole foods for 30 days will influence those parameters.

Excluding frequently sore and cramping muscles, I feel physically good going into this experiment. I wonder if these symptoms are due to lack of creatine since I haven't eaten any red meat for over a month. That will quickly change, as I am off to walk to the butcher in the village to shop for a nice steak for dinner tonight.

Day 4

It is already day four on whole foods and I haven't felt the need to write - probably because I am just loving this food experiment! Finally, I don't feel limited in what I can eat! Partially because of my education as a biologist and health coach, I have a very clear knowledge of what whole foods are, and to the honest, the choices are endless! I have even made some yummy deserts, including a pudding with passion fruit and cream which was divine, or a fresh tangy raspberry, lemon, mint and chia seed sorbet.

Over the last couple of days, I have eaten at least one meal a day with some form of animal protein, including two red meat meals. The physical weakness I felt from not eating meat is gone, so I can exercise intensely again without getting all cramped up. Also, if we want to get into the details of physiological body functions, my intestines are working better than ever before... one big happy dump in the morning... regular, satisfying, perfect!

My period, which is usually extremely regular, was one week late until it finally came on in full force. I am not sure if this unusual irregularity is due to not eating meat for a month or if it is simply attributable to normal pre-menopausal symptoms of a 51-year-old woman.

Day 10

Still going strong on whole foods, although I have experienced a few cravings for sweets or cool mixed cocktail drinks such as gin and tonic. Especially yesterday when Patrick and I walked to our Sunday beach ultimate pickup game. There was a crepe maker on the boardwalk just as we were arriving at the beach and Patrick had a Nutella crepe that looked and smelled absolutely heavenly. Tough!

Even taking into account cravings for junk, this is by far the most pleasant of the four food experiments. Since I can now make whatever I want to eat as long as it's not processed, my love for cooking and desire to try new meals is back in full force. Another advantage of this regime is that there are always options when eating out, such as grilled meat or fish with lemon juice. The thing I miss the most is pasta... maybe I will have to make it myself from whole durum wheat one of these days.

So far the biggest difficulty in my diet this month comes from the fact that I cannot eat any bread that is sold in my favorite bakery close to home, which means that I eat almost no bread (again). But as a whole I am very much enjoying this challenge and starting to be afraid to move on to the next one, where there will be restrictions on things I love to eat once again.

Day 20

I am still going strong on whole foods and am seriously looking forward to a small holiday in the south of Portugal with my family of four, including me of course. It has been great to see how much support I am getting from friends and family on this challenge, which I believe is the easiest one so far. As far as my three homies go, it is fantastic to see them reading labels and ingredient lists, with genuine interest about what is in foods and how to make choices based on what I can eat as well.

For our holiday, we have rented a house in the Algarve for an extended weekend, with a garden and a BBQ. This means we can cook our own whole foods based yummy dinners, based on an amazing menu that Patrick came up with. We all went shopping together and it was great to see that the kids are at this point completely awarene of what whole foods are. Considering how much junk and processed food is out there, it satisfies me to know that my kids can make the choice from a position of knowledge.

Another positive aspect of this challenge is that I have learnt to my own condiments with wholesome ingredients. They taste great and I especially love the homemade mayonnaise (with added garlic or without). I guess the reason I haven't written much is because I am not finding this challenge to be so difficult and therefore feel very little need to vent. On the other hand, I am not losing weight at the rate I thought I would. This may be due to the fact that I am working out regularly and therefore hopefully gaining muscle mass. Also, I can eat a lot of different high calorie foods, such as nuts, that I love.

There is one negative outcome of this food challenge, the sugar cravings. As the weeks go by, I am really missing a little sugary treat… especially when I go to the nearby café, *A Merenda*, where the "pasteis de nata" (Portuguese cream pastries) are absolutely divine.

Day 23

I am now on holiday with the family in a country home close to Tavira in the Algarve. We are all loving the long days on the beach and the late nights of home cooked whole food meals and games with the family. Patrick and I decided to do a "no alcohol" holiday, so no white wine or beer... by I feel a bit like a health nut drinking lots of cold water and yummy foods.

Happily for me, there are two ice-cream houses in Tavira with organic ice-cream (no gluten, lactose, sugar or additives). There is nothing better than enjoying a fresh tasty late afternoon treat while still salty from the beach with my family – no cone allowed though!

Day 30

Wow, Patrick and I got married twenty three years ago today! I am sort of amazed at how happy and in love with each other we still are!

Back to the whole foods experiment at hand, I can't believe it is the last day of the 30 day whole foods challenge. I am afraid of all the ones that are to come, and have no doubt that they will be much tougher for me to complete. And even though I really enjoyed this month, I am very proud that I managed to go 30 days without any refined sugar such as cookies, cakes and chocolate! This is an amazing feat for a sweet tooth such as myself.

My guilty pleasure has been fried potatoes (organic chips and the like). Once more for the sake of transparency, there are some things that I have eaten this month that strictly speaking may not be considered a whole food: vegetable oils (olive oil, coconut oil), wine and beer (only the good stuff, made from fermented grapes or cereals, respectively), table salt (I only use pure sea salt in my cooking, but I have eaten grilled fish and/or meat as well as salads away from home), chips where the ingredients are exclusively potatoes and olive oil. As long as there were no additives or conservatives added, I have chosen to include these as whole foods.

Tomorrow, I will weigh myself and measure my waist before indulging in a sugary treat made from condensed milk, Greek yogurt, and passion fruit that I just prepared and put in the fridge to solidify.

Conclusion

One more month and one more food experiment. Although this one was nowhere near as challenging as the previous ones, or, I am sure, the ones that are to come. In general I loved eating whole foods. Furthermore, unlike with the gluten free or the vegetarian challenge, I felt that I always had an option of something to eat this last month. This may partially explain the result of my weigh-in this morning, which showed my current weight to be at 59.7 Kg, meaning that I lost a measly 200 g in one month without processed sugars or flours. On the other hand, my waist circumference measured at 85 cm, which is 2 cm less than when I started this challenge. Considering that I have been on holiday and have not been playing or practicing ultimate in the last few weeks, this is a positive outcome.

Regarding what it felt like to eat exclusively whole foods, the truth is that the simple fact that I could eat from any food group or macro-nutrient (meat, dairy, fish, vegetables, fruits, whole grains, legumes, fermented foods, etc) stimulated mine and Patrick's love for cooking. This translated into both of us spending a lot of time in the kitchen these last 30 days, and inventing loads of fantastic meals! Since I am a sweet tooth and get sweet cravings, I regularly ate honey, which I sometimes poured over nuts and oats for a treat.

Regarding how I feel physically, I should mention that the tiredness and cramping that I felt so frequently in the last challenge was gone by the first week of this current challenge. My menstrual cycle is regular again, and I feel strong and energized physically as well as mentally. As far as my body and health are concerned, I am now convinced that I need to eat meat or fish to feel my best. Up to now, this was my favorite challenge by a long shot and I am not looking forward to having food limits again.

Positives
- I did not eat junky sugary stuff that I love and did not cheat any time throughout this month (Nutella crepe was tough).
- Learnt a lot about certain foods I thought were whole foods and in fact are not, such as many cheeses (some are less than 50% milk and have starches such as potato starch added), creams

(same as cheese), coconut milk, canned fruits, etc. Reading labels is incredibly important.
- The whole family learnt to read ingredient lists and to discern what is a whole food and what is considered processed or refined.
- I got to seriously appreciate the interest and support that my family and friends are giving me throughout the challenges. In fact, I decided during this challenge that I was going to ask my three homies that live with me to eventually write up a small summary about this experience from their perspective.
- Significantly expanded my capacity for quickly putting together whole food snacks and meals "to go", especially picnics for full days on the beach.
- Lost 2 cm waist circumference and 200 g.

Negatives
- Cutting out sugars and other processed foods did not result in as much difference in my body as I thought it would, perhaps due to less physical activity than usual and the fact that we went on a holiday.
- I probably ate too much good quality cheese as a guilty pleasure.
- Got some serious sugar cravings, especially towards the end of the month.
- Sometimes it was difficult on my family to constantly be forced to eat whole grains instead or white flour products such as pasta, rice or bread.

My day off

Today, I satisfied my humongous desire for high quality Italian ice-cream, which has been off limits due to added sugars. Went to my absolute favored gelato place, called *Santini*, where they make the best fruit and nut gelatos. Oh so yum… I had a huge cone, three flavors, heavenly!

In retrospect

Whenever people ask me which was my favorite of the 12 challenges, this one immediately comes to mind. Not surprisingly, if you think about it, as I could basically eat anything I felt like as long as it did not have processed or refined ingredients. In retrospect, whole foods was also the easiest of the twelve months by far. This is evidenced by the lack of frustrated and unhappy entries in my log. Partially, this can be attributable to the time of year being August, which means the kids had no school and we had some time away as a family on holidays.

Due to my limitations eating out, most of our meals were made and eaten at home, or prepared at home and then taken to the beach. I must, however, mention that we went to an amazing grilled fish smorgasbord in Tavira, where I ate so much fresh grilled fish that I could hardly walk afterwards. Truly amazing! Another highly positive outcome of this month was the desire to go completely clean on our holidays in the South of Portugal, which means that we did not drink alcohol or relish in any other recreational drugs, including refined sugars. I was happy to note that both Patrick and I didn't miss indulging at all!

Whole foods revisited – November 2018

Month four was a huge learning experience for my kids, and I am happy to say, a long lasting one. This does not mean that they only eat whole foods… at 20 and 18 years-old, they both enjoy eating junk at times. They are, however, extremely knowledgeable about what is processed and tend to shy away from eating too much of it. And when they do over-indulge, they feel the negative effects.

Another positive outcome of this challenge was the recognition of how the food industry is intimately linked to the environment, and the realization of the huge cost of mass production/processing/refining on our planet.

Chapter 5 – dairy free

On to challenge number five… no dairy for one month! The reasons I decided to do take dairy products out of my diet are manifold. After the positive experience with the alcohol-free days on holidays last month, I had initially thought to go alcohol free for 30 days. However, I am going to Holland for my brother in law's 50th birthday, and while talking to my mother in law about the possibility of being alcohol free while visiting, she wisely suggested that I take on a different challenge in order to be able to cheer my brother in law at his birthday bash.

To add to that, I am very much aware of the absurd amounts of cheese and yogurt I ate in the last month when doing the whole foods challenge. Third and last, I think this is a valid challenge considering I will be in Holland for over a week and will have to curb devouring amazing Dutch Cheese, quark, and "vla" (a tasty milk based Dutch pudding). To be honest, I think this challenge is going to be very difficult to stick to.

Day 1

I just finished eating a soy yogurt with a slice of quinoa bread and some black berry jam and it was not as bad as I thought it would be. Although I must admit that the whole processing required to get yogurt from soy beans kind of freaks me out. But I did look carefully at the ingredient list, and the ingredients themselves for the natural soy yogurt seemed ok.

But this is not easy! I opened the fridge at least twice today and stared at the cheese. It almost made me cry. I do hope to lose some weight this month and therefore make the sacrifice worth it!

Day 3

Today I decided to treat myself to some high-gluten, fluffy, fresh bread from the corner bakery. I haven't had any in over one month and I really felt like a big fat sandwich. And so I walked over to the local bakery and asked to see the ingredient list for their approximately fifteen different kinds of breads, including carob, rye, whole wheat, spelt, corn, seeds, etcetera. Sadly, they ALL contained dairy in the form of milk powder! There were two that are dairy free on their list, but I have never actually seen them for sale!

Walking a bit further to the supermarket at the village, I did find some dairy free whole wheat bread and had a prosciutto sandwich that tasted most awesome! So far, I am not having as hard a time as I thought I would without dairy. I found some oat milk that I enjoy putting in smoothies and oatmeal, and although I often feel like grabbing for the cheese and/or butter, it's not that bad.

Maybe I'm getting used to having self-imposed limits on what I eat after five months of challenges. On another note, I do have some symptoms that may or may not be related to this challenge. For example, my knees hurt yesterday when I was running around on the sand at beach ultimate practice. Also, after having completely regular intestines for months, I am slightly constipated. Thinking further about this, it is more likely that my intestines are reacting to my going off whole foods and to the re-introduction of crappy preservatives, sugars and additives into my diet again.

Day 7

Admittedly and sadly, I am desperately craving milk products, especially butter and cheese. In fact, I had one of the worse craving days yesterday in a long time, which never ends up well. First thing in the morning, I started eating coconut/egg/sugar cookies, had meat and a beer for lunch, gnocchi for dinner and then a whole pack of milk free cookies at night. Needless to say, my belly is not doing very well this morning. Also, although I decidedly do not like soy yogurt or milk, I did try rice-milk. Not bad, even though I prefer the oat, almond, or coconut milk.

Day 13

Oh my god this is so tough! I have been in Holland for three days to celebrate my brother in law's 50th birthday and I am surrounded by amazing, appetizing, beautiful and oh-so-tasty high-quality dairy products! Throughout the five months of food challenges, I have never been so close to cheating as I am right now. But I knew this was going to be a challenge, especially because I just adore cheese and yogurt and Holland has the best cheeses and yogurts in the world!

Of course, the little devil on my shoulder is constantly whispering in my ear. He seems to be insisting endlessly and saying, "eat whatever you want. Nobody cares about your stupid food challenges." And, "Why are you doing this anyway?" But I can hold strong... even if it's just for me and my self-discipline and self-trust! Interesting that I cannot find any oat milk in Holland, and so have been using coconut-rice milk instead.

Also, I have forgotten to mention what a weakling I have become when it comes to alcohol... one glass of wine or one beer and I am spinning! This is a large difference from my pound-them-back with the boys days! Since we have been here in Holland, I do have one alcoholic beverage every day, which I thoroughly enjoy. Later on tonight is my brother in law's 50th birthday celebration, so let's see how much I drink and party at his hippie themed party.

Day 22

Not eating dairy while in Holland for a week turned out to be an extreme challenge, not only challenging my discipline but also my patience. This is especially the case because it was very clear to me that Dutch dairy foods were, by far, often the best choice of food as far as quality and health goes. Regarding the strong anti-dairy movement currently in the press and advocated by many health professionals, as far as I see it, the Dutch are the perfect example of the wonderful benefits of healthy wholesome dairy. They are generally a very healthy and robust population, and, although I had never noticed before and was really interested to see, the Dutch eat a load of dairy.

I can think of many examples of situations throughout my stay in Holland that show how much dairy the

Dutch eat. Perhaps because of their tendency to eat sandwiches and snacks all day long and have only one hot meal for dinner, it seems to me that dairy is often an opted for food choice in Holland. One afternoon in Patrick's mom hometown, Patrick and I went for lunch with his mom at a healthy sandwich place. It was cool to see that there was only one dairy free option on the entire menu, a humus and grilled vegetable sandwich, which I chose by default and was actually very good. Even on our last night there, dinner was white wine and wonderful finger foods, where the big star was a plate of amazing Dutch cheeses!

To add to these difficult to stay away from dairy experiences in the Netherlands, this last weekend we had a wedding back here in Portugal, and boy did I suffer. Most appetizers had some cheese or cream in them, as did the soup, and over 90% of the deserts. To add insult to injury, I had to avoid the richest and most appetizing cheese table loaded with wonderful, stinky, Portuguese cheeses.

I am proud to say that I have still have not cheated, although I must confess to something which I think is sort of disgusting: I bought butter flavored vegetable spread to put on toast and devoured a couple of slathered toasted slices of bread. Yum and yuck! One of the things I tell my clients not to use is margarine or vegetable spreads, as they are highly processed unnatural foods. But oh well, a little bad is good (happiness is health promoting)and in the end it is what you do 80-90% of the time that counts.

Day 29

Thank goodness that I am almost at the end of this dairy free month. At this point, I am seriously looking forward to digging my teeth into some old Dutch cheeses that we brought back from Holland. I have to admit that the last few days have been a bit of a debauchery when it comes to eating. I bought a large loaf of white "Alentejano" bread, which is like a rustic sower dough bread and is made simply from wheat, salt, water and yeast.

Over the past couple of days, I have been ridiculously feasting on toast or soup with bread cubes. This kind of behavior is no longer normal for me. Also, while hanging out on the couch and watching TV after dinner, Patrick and I have been attacking the licorice that we brought back from Holland. Last week I had lost some weight and was happy with how things were going, especially because I have been practicing disc and working out regularly again... but I have a feeling that this week has been my disgrace. Oh well, that is life, no progress is linear.

Conclusion

These 30 dairy-free days were extremely tough for me, a challenge seriously aggravated by our trip to Holland. Admittedly, I have never been as close to cheating as I have during the last month, and often questioned why I am putting myself through these limitations. At the worst times, the monkeys in my head told me that I am undergoing self-imposed suffering for no reason and should eat whatever I want. Of course, logically I know that the challenges are a good experience, even if in the end, they are just an exercise in self-discipline.

Do I feel differently after not eating dairy for 30 days? Not really. Did it make a huge impact on my diet? Yes! Whereas I often ate a piece of cheese and some nuts when I was hungry, I couldn't... and I missed it terribly. I also missed butter a lot... and not only putting it on toast, but also for cooking.

Regarding my weight, I gained 0.5 kg this month (60.2 kg) and 1 cm in waist circumference (86 cm). This may be simply because I have been overdoing it on crap food the last week and have not been making the healthiest choices, including eating too much white Portuguese bread and cereal with oat milk. Regarding my other body parameters, such as intestinal functioning, menstrual cycle, and sleep, everything appears to be in perfect functioning order.

Positives

- Again, I did not cheat even though it was very difficult, especially while in Holland.
- This month was an educational experience regarding how much of what we eat has "hidden" dairy, including most baked goods and cereals.
- Found that things can be quite tasty without cheese, especially vegetable omelets, pasta and Mexican foods.
- Enjoyed trying different vegetable milks and spreads. Particularly enjoyed oat milk, although I found it a bit too sweet.

- Expanded my cooking with nuts, seeds, and seaweed to make up for the lack of cheese in my recipes.
- Found breakfast alternatives for milk based foods such as smoothie bowls and soft-boiled eggs.
- In general, did not go hungry as there was always a dairy free alternative.
- Maintained excellent energy levels throughout the month.

Negatives
- Missed eating cheese, butter, and yogurt terribly.
- Got some serious sugar and white bread cravings and gave in to these way too often.
- May have gained a bit of weight (although 0.5 kg is not really a gain) and 1 cm on my waist.
- Found it sad to say no to some amazing dairy foods, such as high-quality Dutch cheeses, creamy soups, desserts, etc.

My day off

Today, on my day off, I started the day with a whole foods nut and date bread and a slice of cheese accompanied by a tall glass of cold milk. Later in the day, Patrick and I ate a "pastel de nata" each (wonderful Portuguese cream pastry) with a "dropped" coffee (expresso with a drop of milk) before going for a workout. Also, I ate some great cheeses that we brought from Holland.

Interestingly, I did not feel any discomfort from re-introducing dairy. So no unusual gases, bloating, or any other symptoms. My days off are definitely one of the positive things about these challenges. Today was a heavenly cheesy, milky, creamy day and I feel happy!

In retrospect

Once again, I really enjoyed editing the daily log entries and re-living these first 30 dairy free days. It was an extremely difficult month for me, and I have no doubt that I compensated for the lack of dairy with junky foods. Also, in retrospect, I realize that learning to eat in different ways takes time. Considering the importance and relevance of dairy in my diet normally, this was a significant month. I am sure that I learnt a lot this month about cooking without dairy or how to make the right snack choices.

As important as dairy was, and is, in my diet, the truth is that this was the first month of a total of five dairy free months over a one year period. After completing the other four still upcoming consecutive dairy free challenges (dairy and gluten free, macrobiotic, paleolithic diet and vegan), I got so used to not having dairy that it didn't even cross my mind as a food choice. Today, almost two weeks after the challenges are over, I eat dairy on a regular basis, especially Greek yogurt with nuts and fruits, stinky and highly fermented cheeses, and butter in my recipes.

No dairy revisited – November 2018

Just the other day, I looked in the fridge to see at least 7 different types of cheese… along with the butter, milk and natural Greek yogurt that this family considers part of our "staple foods". We eat a lot of dairy in our house, and both kids drink a lot of milk. Do I think that is health? I don't think it is unhealthy, as long as we also eat a lot of fresh plant based foods. I do think quality counts, and therefore make sure to buy dairy products from happy cows, ones that graze.

Chapter 6 – alcohol free

I realized at some point in the last month that I have been able to drink alcohol throughout all my challenges so far. In fact, alcohol has often turned out to be the "go to" option at social gatherings, when my limitations did not allow me to eat most or any of what was being served. It is gluten free, coffee free, vegetarian, good beer and wine are whole foods, and it has no dairy. So now I feel that I can only gain from going one month without alcohol.

To be honest, I don't think this challenge will be too difficult. One of the main reasons I decided to do this is that after five months of food limitations, I feel the need to have a month that I can eat anything that I want. This is especially the case when I think about the radical food regime that I will be doing next month for the toughest challenge so far – number seven. But first, let's now see how alcohol free goes.

Day 1

I decided to start this challenge with a mini liquid detox, and therefore to eat only fruit and vegetables in liquid form for 36 hours. This means that for the time period starting last night before going to bed on night one, the entire day today, and a second night tonight, I can only eat fruit and vegetable smoothies and creamed vegetable soups.

Although the beginning of the day went well, by late afternoon I felt very tired and lacking in energy at now at night-time I have a dull headache at the back of my head. These symptoms may or may not be related to lack of calories. Regarding the alcohol free challenge itself, I did feel like an ice-cold beer in the afternoon while walking on the beach with my man, but nothing too difficult to overcome.

Day 2

I weighed in this morning and lost 0.5 kg in one day with my mini-detox. After eating a huge plate of oatmeal with nuts and raisins for breakfast, I got back my full energy levels, and already worked out, went for a long walk, and am right now actively working. But, I still can't get rid of the nagging headache at the back of my head.

Day 3

After feeling decently well in the morning yesterday, I spent the entire rest of the day nursing a wicked headache, as well as feeling nauseous and with an upset stomach. I must have gone for a dump (not diarrhea) about ten times in the last 24 hours and lost another 300 grams even though I have been eating normally.

Not sure if it was the 36-hour detox, the re-introduction of dairy, or a virus. Today I have a bit of a stuffy nose, so it could very well be a virus. I did go to practice last night and felt ok energy-wise running around on the sand.

Day 6

Boy, I have never been as close to cheating in these challenges as I was this last weekend. It was very tough indeed! The reason being that we had a close friend, who lives in the UK and enjoys good wine and cold beer, staying with us for a few nights. It was oh-so-tough to watch him and Patrick enjoy great red wines while catching up as I sipped some herbal infusion.

To add insult to injury, we also had the last day of the National Ultimate beach ultimate league in which my team played 4 easily won games with a bunch of great beer drinking players. Man-oh-man... during the closing ceremonies, I actually felt pain in my chest and abdomen just thinking how good a cold beer would taste. I hung in there, but barely!

Day 13

Although I often get desires for a cold beer, a cold glass of white wine, or a gin and tonic, on a day to day basis this challenge is reasonably easy compared to the other ones. That being said, it is kind of funny how close I have been to cheating the few times that I am in a social situation in which everyone around me is drinking.

The social aspect of drinking also has made me realize how difficult it must be for those who can't consume alcohol. For example, I went to the theatre with girlfriends from my book-club and felt a bit like a fundamentalist drinking sparkling water while everyone else was drinking wine during the break.

Day 18

Another very difficult weekend without falling off the wagon. I am actually curious about where that phrase comes from and am going to google it now, back in a second.

Ok, found something that quenches my curiosity. According to google, the saying "falling off the wagon" supposedly originated in the late 19th century during the time of the Prohibition. It refers to men not going to the water wagon to quench their thirst, and choosing to drink alcoholic beverages instead of water (https://english.stackexchange.com/questions/37132/origin-of-the-idiom-falling-off-the-wagon).

I'm glad I looked that up, it actually makes more sense than I thought, since I always imagined that you needed to be drunk to fall off the wagon, making the saying nonsensical to me. Anyway, this last weekend was again a true test in discipline and will power, and I repeat, it was hard not to fall off the water wagon.

First, we had my niece's birthday party on Saturday night. Approximately 70 semi-intoxicated teenagers and a load of tasty and happy drinks… but not for me. And that is not all, this one was a double whammy! The day after the party, I played at the first women's beach ultimate tournament in Portugal on Sunday. AAARGHHHH…. I suffered a lot!

One of the players who has been in Portugal for a few years and is going back to Germany, brought some great German beers to the field to cheer with the ladies. Oh man… I could only look, cheer the ladies with my water, and try not to weep from a self-imposed safe distance.

I hate not being able to do what I feel like! AAARRGGHHH!!!!

Day 21

Today, I am starting to believe that this alcohol-free challenge is having a positive effect on me. I am extremely clear headed and strong and happy not to have cheated, not only in this current challenge but also for the last six months. Interestingly, I am also getting used to not drinking where I normally loved to do so. For example, last week at the book-club dinner with the ladies, where I usually drink copious amounts of wine, it was strangely and unexpectedly easy to stay wine-free. Hurray for that! Now, I am beginning to fear the next challenge, where the food limitations will be again a part of my daily life.

Day 25

The alcohol free 30 days are almost at an end and I am still not sure if I will have the capacity to do the diet regime that I planned to do next. I think I may be getting cold feet about what is to come. But one thing is for sure, I am really enjoying how I feel and how these challenges are empowering me to explore different foods and drinks.

Day 30

Here is the day, the last alcohol-free day! To be honest, I am more worried about if and how I will be able to do what I wanted to do as the seventh challenge than I am looking forward to having a drink.

Conclusion

On a day to day basis, being alcohol free was by far the easiest challenge of all the challenges so far. With that in mind, it was also the challenge that I came closest to cheating, particularly in three or four social situations where I just felt I "needed" a drink. I decided to take the almost physical pain I felt because I couldn't drink as a sign, and have therefore decided to decrease the amount of alcohol I ingest.

Considering that I don't drink daily, this means less booze on party nights. Also interesting, I got used to and started enjoying having a clear head, especially at social get togethers when everyone around proceeded to get fuzzy. I am now curious to see how my alcohol consumption will change on a long-term perspective.

Regarding my weight, I lost 0.6 kg this month (59.6 kg) as well as decreased 3 cm in waist circumference (83 cm). Not sure if the weight loss is completely alcohol related, as I am slowly getting back to my before-quitting-smoking weight of almost three years ago. Also, I find that I make healthier food choices and hand myself over to cravings less often if I have no restrictions. The waist circumference, however, is most likely at least partially alcohol related. Funny enough, today is my day off and I probably will not drink any alcohol. Actually curious to see how I will feel when I do...

Positives

- Again, I did not cheat even though I had a few close moments.
- Loved the fact that I could eat anything I felt like eating, especially after some months of food limitations.
- After overcoming moments of frustration, I started to enjoy feeling clear headed as everyone around me got fuzzy at parties.
- Found that great meals are just as nice with sparkling water and lemon.
- Enjoyed trying different homemade fruit and spice water infusions.
- Lost some weight and 3 cm waist circumference.

Negatives

- At parties and social gatherings, I often felt like a teetotaler (which means someone who abstains, or advocates abstaining, from alcohol - it is worth reading the origins of this word, try looking it up on Wikipedia).
- Missed out on tasting some excellent wines.
- Missed my occasional sunset drinks with my husband at the beach (although herbal tea was nice too).

My day off

Funny enough, I didn't drink any alcohol on my day off. Feeling powerful and clear headed and not necessarily needing or wanting a drink. Next challenge will allow me to have one single glass of white wine once or twice a week, but that will be it as far as drinks go for a while!

In retrospect

One thing is for sure, over the food-challenges year I seem to have lost the capacity to drink the way I used to. I still love my gin and tonics, good wines and cold beers, but one or two drinks and I am floating nicely… and quickly start feeling unpleasantly tipsy if I drink too much. This change is likely due to a bunch of factors, including weight loss, healthy eating, and, I would say mostly because of generally drinking a lot less and therefore lack of drink training.

This alcohol-free month was not the first time going dry over the last few years. Before the world beach ultimate championships in Dubai in 2015, I did not touch alcohol or recreational drugs for 5 months. Also interesting is the reaction that I had after the 36-hour detox, including an upset stomach and headache, which is reminiscent to the first days of my intermittent fasting challenge in month 12.

No alcohol revisited – November 2018

I would like to take the opportunity to share some recent results on alcohol consumption and health. Alcohol has been consumed for thousands of years. It was the drink of choice in some cultures such as the Romans, where the fermented wine had an important role in safe hydration.

A recent publication published in The Lancet this summer

(https://www.thelancet.com/journals/lancet/article/PIIS

0140-6736(18)31310-2/fulltext) looks at the Global Burden of disease of alcohol intake. Their results have been picked up by the press to state that alcohol is mostly detrimental at any level. However, the authors show that alcohol at low levels (one bottle of wine or less per week) protects against cardiac diseases. Also, there is no data provided regarding the type of alcohol that is being consumed. In my opinion, measuring grams of alcohol per a time period fails to take into account important data.

There is no arguing that fermented alcoholic drinks like wine and beer have strong health promoting properties, including probiotics and anti-oxidants. Wine consumption has often been associated with longevity, and an important part of cultures with good health metrics, such as the Mediterranean.

Besides physical health, the pleasure we get from enjoying a drink with friends is so important! It is when we use alcohol as a crutch that there is a problem, or as a place to hide. No disrespect to those who cannot drink alcohol, and by no means is alcohol a must for a complete fulfilled life. But for me, moderation counts... and I do enjoy a drink and sometimes many drinks but I want to be lucid for the grand majority of the time.

Chapter 7 – ketogenic diet

After half a year of self-imposed food limitations, I feel ready as well as slightly anxious to start the seventh consecutive 30-day challenge, the ketogenic diet. There are a bunch of reasons I chose to do this regime at this time, but before I get into that let me describe the ketogenic diet and what it entails.

I have been somewhat afraid of this diet, as it is, by far, the most radical of all the challenges I have done. The whole concept behind the ketogenic diet is that a diet high in fat and low in carbs as well as low in protein results in the body adapting to utilize fat instead of glucose for energy, through a process called ketosis.

Considering the shift that the body and brain must undergo to use fat instead of glucose for energy, the ketogenic diet has a strong impact on the body as well as the brain. This diet has been used for over a century to manage seizures in patients with epilepsy, and sometimes works to control epileptic episodes in those who do not respond to pharmacological approaches.

Lately, this diet has gotten a lot of attention from sports aficionados and athletes as a tool to re-shape the body, augment lean body mass (lose body fat), and influence endurance. Before we get into how to eat on the ketogenic diet, I must bore you a little with the biology. Hang in there, and if you are truly not interested in the "why and how" of the crazy month to come, then feel free to skip the next two paragraphs. Here we go.

The whole concept of fat adaptation is based on the fact that although our bodies and brains preferentially use carbs for energy, we have a much more limited amount of stored carbohydrate in our bodies than we do stored fat. The absolute maximum amount of carbs that our bodies can store (mostly in the form of glycogen stored in muscles and the liver) is 15 g per kg of body weight, with the average being closer to 500 g of stored carbs per person. This, at 4 calories per gram, translates into 2000 calories of stored carbs. Compare that to anywhere between 7-30 % of our body mass of fat (or more for so many overweight people) stored in the form of triglycerides. At 9 calories per gram of fat, this means that a very lean 60 kg person with 10 % body fat has 54 000 calories of stored fat in their body.

The much larger amount of energy available from stored fat taken together with the adaptive capacity of our body to use fat for energy supposedly results in a significant increase in long-term energy levels. In truth, our bodies often use fat for energy, such as in the morning after a low-carb meat and salad dinner, or when we fast for approximately 24 hours (or less if we are physically active).

In today's much publicized diets and lifestyles, there is a tendency to label very low carb diets as ketogenic diets. However, in a strict ketogenic diet, protein content must also be strictly controlled, as protein is quickly converted into glucose for our body to use for energy. For this month, I opted to go on a strict ketogenic diet, following the guidelines often administered to epileptic patients.

This means that I will be ingesting less than 50 g of carbs a day (in the form of "over the ground" vegetables and some fruits), 1 g of protein per kg of body weight (in my case approximately 60 g of protein per day), and the rest of my daily calories in fat. If we do the math for a 2000 calorie a day diet, this means that I eat less than 200 calories in carbs, 240 calories in protein, and approximately 1600 calories in fat per day. Converting fat calories to grams, at 9 calories per gram, means 178 g of fat per day. That translates into a decent block of fat a day, more than one third of a pound! Yuk!

Just the thought of eating this much fat without some starch to soak it up or protein to dilute it is making me slightly nauseous. Anyway, in the end, I am consciously choosing to go through with this. You may, as I have often done myself, question me as to why I am doing this particular challenge. I am not sure why, but perhaps because it is so different from my high grain diet. Or and also, perhaps because I am curious as to how the metabolic changes will impact my energy levels and/or thinking speed.

Also, as strange as it sounds, I think eating tons of fat may do something to help me to lose a couple of kilos that have accumulated around my waist in the last few years. I have to admit, I am not looking forward to eating so much fat for a month, although I am curious to see how it goes.

Day 3

Three days of this new challenge have gone by and I

am surprised that I still haven't had an alcoholic drink. Regarding the ketogenic diet itself, after a few days of eating loads of stinky high fat cheese, avocados, eggs cooked in butter, meat and cream, I am starting to think that this may not have been the wisest choice.

It is interesting that I am not hungry at all. Quite the contrary, I feel constantly full and slightly nauseous. This is probably due to the specifics of fat digestion, which is very different to how we digest carbs or proteins and is generally a more prolonged process. Also, I am very surprised at how regular my intestines are... which is a good thing! Now going off to the market to buy some high fat stuff to cook, wish me luck!

Day 5

This entry marks the historical day where Donald Trump was elected the president of the United States. Oh my... I slept like crap because Patrick kept waking me up telling me Trump was ahead. When I did come upstairs in the morning, Tomas, our son, told me that he woke up at sunrise to his dad yelling at the TV while the final results were being announced. I went for a walk with my mom, but I can't seem to accept that this actually happened, I feel like the world has had a lobotomy. Hopefully writing here will distract me from this insane political and societal cluster f**k and get my energies and mind onto the things that I can control, namely food.

The truth is that after five days of eating a lot of fat and very little carbs (and limited protein) I am starting to feel a difference in my metabolism. Thankfully, the initial sick feeling I used to get just by thinking about eating fats is gone and I am surprisingly able to enjoy fatty meal after fatty meal.

Thank goodness I am highly creative in the kitchen. Today I made pancakes with eggs and homemade walnut flour for breakfast and ate them with black berries. They were very good. For lunch, I had a green salad full of shrimp and mayo which also tasted great.

All in all, I am never hungry and have a load of mental energy. Also, my intestines are working great. So, right now, all is good. Whereas a couple of days ago I thought I would never be able to do this diet for the entire month, at this point I feel confident that I will. I must be careful about what I choose to do in the 30 days afterwards to make sure I don't shock my system too much.

Day 11

After a positive period feeling great on the ketogenic diet (keto), I am once again just hanging in there. This is quite the radical diet and is not easy to follow at all. Amazing that after almost two weeks eating fat, I am still enjoying my fatty meals. So eating itself is not the problem for me.

The last days have been mediocre, I have been getting highly creative in the kitchen so that I can continue to enjoy eating the limited amounts of foods that I can eat. Lots of cheese, eggs, fatty meats, fatty fishes, nuts (some nuts, such as high carb pistachios and cashews are out), high fat yogurt, avocados, and greens.

Although I don't believe in frequently weighing myself,

this diet has just gotten me so curious that I had to weigh in, and found that I have lost 1 kg in 11 days. Considering that I am not hungry at all, exercising very little and eating a load of fat, I am shocked.

I have no desire to exercise. At this point I have an overwhelming lack of general energy and get somewhat nauseous when I try to push myself. I also notice that I am much lazier than usual after dark. There has been a serious stomach flu going around, which both my son and husband fell victims to, so that may explain some of the "keto flu" symptoms that have turned me into a couch potato the last few nights.

Besides actively walking around during the day and a few bouts of intense 15 minute workouts, I have been very sluggish and have done very little. Tonight, I am going to play disc on the beach and am curious as to how I will feel.

Day 12

I didn't make it to practice last night because I felt that my muscles were extremely tired and weak... to the point that it was almost painful. Partially in response to my physical lethargy and partially due to my science mind, I decided to review the scientific literature discussing the effects of the ketogenic diet on athletic performance and brain function (see reviews and references at the end of this chapter).

This post may therefore be a bit of a science lesson. If you are not interested in the fatty science, again, I apologize and suggest you skip this entry completely. If you are interested, and I hope that you are, then read on... I will try to make it worth your time.

From what I have read after much browsing and researching, there is no doubt that the ketogenic diet influences body composition and results in weight loss. From the perspective of sports, the physical adaptive requirements and responses that influence athletic performance vary greatly depending on the type of sport, as you can see by the obvious differences between the body of an elite marathon runner compared to that of a wrestler or a heavy weight lifter.

The ketogenic diet seems to have no significant effects (some publications show slightly positive, some slightly negative and others no effects)Regarding on long-term aerobic endurance, such as that required for marathon running. Conversely, the majority of studies show that the ketogenic diet imposes negative effects on anaerobic "explosive" performance, mostly attributed to decreased glycogen storage in muscles and therefore limited capacity for anaerobic muscle contraction.

These results help make sense of how my body feels as well as are in accordance with my current knowledge and another relevant factor that I have read a lot about over the last few days. The factor of the "perceived effort" by the athlete, which plays a significant role in athletic performance and seems to be negatively augmented by lack of available carbohydrates.

If you are interested in food and athletic performance and would like to read further, I suggest taking a look at a Joint Position published by the Dietitians of Canada and the American College of Sports Medicine. Their comprehensive review of the literature clearly indicates that what is best for athletic performance is a whole foods diet rich in vitamins, minerals and nutrients. Furthermore, they also show which nutrition adjustments are most effective just before, during and after intense training or competition for various forms physical demands as well as numerous times of exertion.

Contrary to the effects, or lack of effects, of the ketogenic diet on athletic performance, there is strong evidence of the positive effects of this diet on other physical parameters, and especially on brain health. For example, the ketogenic diet is known to provide neuroprotective effects on patients with Parkinson's, Alzheimer, or those that have suffered brain injury.

Also, when applied for a limited time, the classical ketogenic diet has positive effects on not alcoholic fatty liver disease and on reducing the levels of triglycerides in the blood. Which brings me to an interesting point, I am shocked at how many people think eating fat is what causes high blood fat and high cholesterol, including many health professionals.

It is currently known that the fat in our blood is mostly attributable to fat produced by our livers rather than ingested fat, and a significant proportion of the fat that our livers make comes from excess carbs that are not burned up by our body's energetic needs. Because so many people have been telling me that my cholesterol is going be crazy high due to my eating so much fat, I have decided get my blood lipid profile (cholesterol test) done at the end of this challenge.

Day 13

Almost at the end of the second week on the ketogenic diet and I continue to feel very tired, especially at the end of the day. In fact, the muscle fatigue is constant, to the point that I have a constant dull pain in my legs. Taken together with what I read about the ketogenic diet causing mineral imbalances due to loss of body water (hypo-magnesium, calcium, potassium, and sodium), I bought some multi-vitamins and minerals and started taking them today. Later this afternoon, I will do a work out and then later go to disc practice.

Day 14

Today, I am finally feeling a little bit better. What a relief, maybe I am finally getting keto-adapted. I do, however, have a headache, which I am not sure is related to this diet regime. It could simply be because I have my period, the atmospheric pressure (I am sensitive to this and it is a dreary grey day) or a virus.

Yesterday, I was an absolute mess! I cancelled going to disc practice at the last minute because even simple walking tired me out. Normally on Thursdays I do volunteer work at the community center about a mile from home, and enjoy exploring different paths when walking back home.

This was not the case yesterday, when the journey home felt impossibly long and I felt like an old and haggard lady as I dragged my feet all the way home. Worse than that, I kept fretting about how long it was taking to get to the next viewed milestone such as the pedestrian bridge I can see from some distance. The whole walk, which is usually a pleasure, was a serious chore.

To add to that, I was edgy and impatient all day. I seriously considered cutting this experiment short. Thanks to a lot of encouragement and support from Patrick and my accountability coach, I am glad I hung in there.

Day 15

I decided to stop taking the vitamin and mineral supplementation, since they did not seem to help after taking them for two days. The lack of energy and lack of desire to move mean that although I have been actively doing basic maintenance activities around the house (grocery shopping, walking to do chores, cleaning up the house, etcetera), I have not done any serious exercise this week. In fact, I have done very little physical activity this entire challenge.

On another note, I read an interesting fact about this diet regarding weight loss which I think is important to share with those choosing to do this to lose weight. It does require me to get a little into biology, I hope you are getting used to it.

Recall the earlier discussion about carbs stored in the body in the form of glycogen? Well, this stored glycogen, which is typically close to 500 g in an adult, is associated with water at a 1:2 or 1:3 ratio in our muscles and our liver. As glycogen stores get depleted after some time without eating carbs, there is quick initial weight loss due to the glycogen being used up and the consequent loss of the water water associated with the used up glycogen.

This means that up to 1.5 kg of weight loss in the first week can be attributed to glycogen and associated water being depleted rather than burning body fat. No wonder I feel like a raisin and look like crap! It will be interesting to see how the rest of the month goes and how quickly my weight resumes back to normal afterwards.

Day 17

Still hanging in there. Once again, getting creative in the kitchen so that I am not eating the same thing all the time. Made a "dessert" consisting of full fat cream, a quarter of a pomegranate and some plain bone gelatin. Tasted great with some high fat walnuts. Also, I went to the butcher and bought a large bone to boil up with some veggies to make a nice salty high mineral broth. Although I am still weak, I am starting to feel a lot better. After so many failed attempts, today I may I have the strength to work out, finally! Let's see how it goes.

Day 18

Last night, I did a short, 3-part intense exercise routine (thanks David Pimenta) which includes burpees, push-ups, V-ups and squats, and felt almost normal. Also, as far as cooking and eating goes, I am starting to adventure more with unsweetened coconut to get away from the fatty dairy. Still 12 days to go, but I think I will be able to stick with it. Tonight I will most likely go to play disc after some weeks off, and I am curious as to how I will feel running on the sand.

Day 19

Getting a bit more used to the diet and feeling less tired at the end of the day. Disc was cancelled last night, so I still haven't played or practiced since being on a ketogenic diet. I do feel strange sometimes, a bit dizzy and nauseous. Not enjoying this one.

Day 24

After three and a half weeks eating tons of fat, I am finally feeling my energetic self again! This is a good change from this last weekend, when I was again seriously thinking of giving up this crazy diet. I felt weak, unmotivated, sick of eating fat and was badly craving carbs, especially healthy whole grain carbs.

But again, with the help of great friends, I managed to get over the hump. First, we had dinner with Moi and Inês, who is an amazing cook and prepared the most incredible ketogenic dinner, consisting of a slow roasting pork shoulder and lots of fantastic fatty chesses. Heavenly! Second, at Patrick's suggestion, I have decided to add a new challenge "within a challenge" to this last week - I will work out hard every day to test how I feel and to see if it makes an impact on losing accumulated body fat.

Yesterday, I finally went to play disc. Although I felt quite dizzy at times and had to stop for a few moments, I could run on the sand and catch. Throwing was tougher as my arms felt rubbery and weak and my balance was a bit out of whack.

The good news is that I feel committed and strong in my resolution to end this with a bang. Later on today, I will do a powerful weights and cardio routine at home. My weight has maintained at 1 kg less than when I started this challenge.

Day 29

I have had it with this diet, and want to quit now! Amazing that there is only one more day to go and I am nevertheless struggling to hang in there.

Since today is Friday, I decided to get my blood work done this morning on an empty stomach. What an adventure that turned out to be! Right after waking up, I walked over to the local pharmacy on an empty stomach after an overnight fast for the blood tests. The result for my total blood cholesterol was 290 mg/dL, which is a little high, but within my normal parameters. However, the result for the blood triglycerides levels of 375 mg/dL was ridiculously high... butter in my veins!

I walked back home quite unhappy at this unexpected result, especially after spending an entire month insisting that as unhealthy as this diet was, it was not going to raise my blood lipids. Pissed off and eating my ketogenic breakfast of full fat Greek yogurt and walnuts, I realized that the triglyceride level was impossible! Especially considering that I typically have low triglyceride concentrations in my blood. Furiously, off I ran back to the pharmacy, now on a full stomach, and asked the pharmacist to repeat the test. She told me that since I had just eaten, my results would only be higher, and that my triglyceride results were not surprising since I had been eating fat for a month. So I made a deal with her, if the results of the second test were worse or the same, I would pay for the test again. However, if not, then she would refund my original 6 Euros. She agreed, and the second test resulted in a triglyceride measure of 199 mg/dL! Almost half of the initial test, and now with food in my belly and triglycerides quickly on the way from my digestive tract into my blood. Urghhh!

I did get my money back, but the whole experience was quite unsettling for me. Especially because it obviously indicated that the results of the blood work were completely unreliable and therefore meant absolutely nothing! I hate crap data!

After bitching to Patrick about the whole thing, he suggested that I go to an accredited medical clinic and get the whole blood work properly re-done, even though I had eaten. Off I ran to the analysis clinic. I ran in and "almost rudely" insisted with the nurse to take my blood quickly to avoid my recently eaten meal to influence the results. The nurse tried to talk me out of paying for the test, as my values would be off due to having eaten and would mean nothing.

In the end, I won, and the results I got were mostly comparable to my normal levels from previous analysis. These were 290 mg/dL in total cholesterol (compared to 254 in 2015), 92 mg/dL in HDL (compared to 85), 174 mg/dL LDL (compared to 150) and 120 mg/dL triglycerides (compared to 84). And this, about one hour after eating a high fat meal. I like to think that this is what justifies the slight increase in the level of my triglycerides, and in turn, total blood cholesterol.

Day 30

Last day, thank goodness! Hanging in there and not eating much today. Looking forward to a large bowl of oatmeal tomorrow!

Conclusion

This was, by a long shot, the most difficult and radical of all the food challenges so far, and the one that I needed the most support to not call it quits. For this, I must thank Patrick (my husband) for pushing me to start pushing my body physically even though I felt so tired, as well as my Health Coach, Patricia, for supporting me and incentivizing me to stick with it.

I learnt a lot this month about foods and diets. Also, I read a load of science on ketosis and its effects on the body and brain. In the end, although it was very difficult, I now consider that 2-4 weeks on a ketogenic diet to be a true detox (I like the term ketox).

The "purging" aspect from this diet comes from the fact that when in ketosis, the body is forced to utilize and therefore renew fat stores, something that rarely happens when there are carbs available to meet bodily energy needs. Also, there is something about a keto adapted brain, or a brain that is adapted to getting its energy to function from fat. As bad as my body has felt, my brain has been sharp and on.

This has not been a great month as far as exercise is concerned. Excluding the last week, where I pushed myself to work out and to play disc, I didn't do much physical activity and felt weak and tired all the time. Regarding weight loss and waist circumference, I lost 2 kg between the first and last day of the diet (weighing in at 57.6 kg) and 1 cm waist circumference (82 cm). Keep in mind, this weight loss can at least partially be attributed to loss of water from my body. In fact, I have felt dehydrated many times this month, regardless of how much water I drank or salt/minerals I ate.

Positives

- What a learning experience this month was! I often felt that I was my own lab rat and both the scientist and the subject of a crazy experiment. In the end, I am proud to have stuck with it.
- I got highly creative shopping for and cooking with high fat foods, and made fun recipes and soups that were enjoyable even when the whole idea of eating fat made me nauseous.
- I slept great throughout the entire month and maintained regular bowel movements.
- It was very interesting to feel the physical effects of ketogenic adaptation. For me, it took about three weeks to feel normal and somewhat physically powerful.
- My brain function seemed to improve. I felt very sharp, quick thinking and creative.
- Lost some weight, although at least 1 kg is only water.
- Detoxed. I have come to the conclusion that this diet is highly anti-inflammatory and a good shock

to the system when done at the right time and in the right way. It is likely that I do a ketogenic eating bout periodically on myself throughout my life.

Negatives
- For the first three weeks, I felt very weak and had no physical energy for exercise.
- I felt nauseous many times, and got sick of eating fat.
- Although there were always options of something to eat, this diet is oftentimes very limiting and often unpalatable.
- I found this diet extremely difficult to do and maintain.

My day off

I am oh-so-glad to be eating normally again. Happily, I don't feel at all like junk food. Rather, today I am relishing in whole grains, fruits, and sweet potatoes.

Afternote (February 7th, 2017): A cousin who is also a close friend of mine suffers from "cluster headaches", and has episodes of nightly incapacitating headaches for periods of time that can last up to five months. In desperation and on my suggestion, he tried the ketogenic diet.

Interestingly, after three days he started to notice changes that are typically associated with breaks in the cycles of headaches, such as variation in the time of day the headaches set in (in his case in the middle of the night changing to around dinner time) and alterations in their intensity.

After one week, he finally had one pain-free night. Due to the difficulty in maintaining this diet long-term, he did not continue the ketogenic diet, but I thought this experience was worth the mention.

In retrospect

The ketogenic challenge was not an easy chapter to edit. Although I could tell that my brain was on by the quality of my writing needing little adjustment, I am right now slightly nauseated just from reliving the experience. It was not easy an easy 30 days! On the other hand, it was a huge learning experience and probably the challenge that I learnt the most from out of the entire year.

Looking back now, I think this was the month that had the biggest impact on my body and mind. It was also the challenge that inspired me to keep going on this food anthropological journey, since after being able to stick to this way of eating for 30 days I felt that I could take on any food challenge.

Regarding the long-term effects of eating 75 % of my caloric intake from fat for 30 days, I now believe this experiment influenced my metabolism and that my body is currently better adapted to burning fat. I often eat "keto friendly" very low carb and high fat meals, especially as the first and/or last meals of the day or on days like today that I am mostly focused on the book and therefore doing very little physical activity.

In sum, I will apply what I learnt this month throughout

my life. It is unlikely that I will do a strict ketogenic diet as drastically or for as long as I did this month, but am now a full believer in the physical and mental health promoting properties of a periodic "ketox-detox" reset. This month was a lesson on how resilient our bodies are, having an incredible capacity of adaption to very different energy sources. From a physical and psychological perspective, I am convinced that having undergone this experience helped me adjust quicker to the intermittent fasting 30-day challenge that I did on month twelve.

The ketogenic diet revisited – November 2018

It is now two years since I did this challenge, and it maintains the challenge that I learnt the most about our metabolism. Over the last few years, I have enjoyed seeing the press grab fat by the horns and talking about it as a healthy food option.

The latest issue of Science magazine, a special issue on diet and health, was published two days ago. In it, there is an extensive review entitled Dietary fat: From foe to friend? By Ludwig et al (2018). The science is extensive and important, with the following points of consensus shown (copied verbatim and worth reading carefully, as each point is loaded with info):

1. With a focus on nutrient quality, good health and low chronic disease risk can be achieved for many people on diets with a broad range of carbohydrate-to-fat ratios.

2. Replacement of saturated fat with naturally occurring unsaturated fats provides health benefits for

the general population. Industrially produced trans fats are harmful and should be eliminated. The metabolism of saturated fat may differ on carbohydrate-restricted diets, an issue that requires study.

3. Replacement of highly processed carbohydrates (including refined grains, potato products, and free sugars) with unprocessed carbohydrates (nonstarchy vegetables, whole fruits, legumes, and whole or minimally processed grains) provides health benefits.

4. Biological factors appear to influence responses to diets of differing macronutrient composition. People with relatively normal insulin sensitivity and β cell function may do well on diets with a wide range of carbohydrate-to-fat ratios; those with insulin resistance, hypersecretion of insulin, or glucose intolerance may benefit from a lower-carbohydrate, higher-fat diet.

5. A ketogenic diet may confer particular metabolic benefits for some people with abnormal carbohydrate metabolism, a possibility that requires long-term study.

6. Well-formulated low-carbohydrate, high-fat diets do not require high intakes of protein or animal products. Reduced carbohydrate consumption can be achieved by substituting grains, starchy vegetables, and sugars with nonhydrogenated plant oils, nuts, seeds, avocado, and other high-fat plant foods.

7. There is broad agreement regarding the fundamental components of a healthful diet that can serve to inform policy, clinical management, and individual dietary choice. Nonetheless, important questions relevant to the epidemics of diet-related chronic disease remain. Greater investment in nutrition

research should assume a high priority.

I would argue in point two that the origin of the saturated fat is an important piece of data when it comes to analyzing the health effects of saturated fats. Many populations thrive on saturated fats from plant sources, like the coconut. Another source of saturated fat is meats, and no doubt we should decrease our production of large animals for food, especially for the sake of our planet. Industrially produced saturated fats (typically from plant oils) are to be avoided, as are all non-naturally occurring foods.
It is clear from the above points that although we know a lot, there is still a great amount to be learnt. Point 3 is worth the mention, considering that it about carbohydrates and the importance of whole grains and other edible plants. This shows the importance of the whole of what we eat, rather than the specifics. Foods in a meal interact through digestion, and thereby affect the digestion process.

References

Dietitians of Canada: Nutrition and Athletic Performance: https://www.dietitians.ca/Dietitians-Views/Specific-Populations/Nutrition-and-Athletic-Performance.aspx

Gasior M, Rogawski MA, Hartman AL 2006. Neuroprotective and disease-modifying effects of the ketogenic diet. Behavioural Pharmacology, Vol. 17, pp.

431

Helge JW. 2002. Long-term fat diet adaptation effects on performance, training capacity, and fat utilization. Medicine and Science in Sports and Exercise, Vol. 34, pp. 1499

Rebecca CS, Crawford PA. 2012. Low-carbohydrate ketogenic diets, glucose homeostasis, and nonalcoholic fatty liver disease. Current Opinion in Clinical Nutrition and Metabolic Care, Vol. 15, pp. 374

Thomas DT, Erdman KA, Burke LM. 2016. Position of the Academy of Nutrition and Dietetics, Dietitians of Canada, and the American College of Sports Medicine: Nutrition and Athletic Performance. Journal of the Academy of Nutrition and Dietetics, Vol. 116, pp. 501

Ludwig DS, Willett WC, Volek JS, Neuhouser ML. 2018 Dietary fat: From foe to friend? Science, Vol. 362, pp. 764

Chapter 8 – gluten and dairy free

Onto the eighth consecutive food challenge, no dairy and no gluten for 30 days! I am elated that the previous challenge has come to an end and am almost giddy at the thought of eating carbs as a regular part of my diet again! After one month on the extremely hard to stick to ketogenic diet, I think this month will be a breeze.

Funny how things change... how we change. In this case, my unexpected positive mind frame is a pleasant surprise, especially considering how difficult it was for me to do each of these two limitations separately in the not so distant past. Shows how our perception of what is easy or difficult is relative to our experiences. After last month, this seems like a breeze!

I weighed myself this morning just to make sure that I keep track of weight changes for each challenge and weighed in at 58.6 kg. I was not surprised to have gained back one of the two kilograms that I had lost last month, probably due to replenishing the carbohydrates on my day off, and therefore gaining back body storages of glycogen as well as the water associated with these.

This morning, my first bowl of oatmeal tasted like heaven! To meet the current challenge, it made with vegetable milk, half a banana, rolled oats, seeds and cinnamon. After 24 hours of eating carbs, I feel completely different. My hair is shinier, my skin suppler, and my physical energy levels much higher. I am looking forward to this month, and to cutting out the cheeses and creams which I have been eating in excess for the last 30 days.

Day 3

As expected after a complete month on the ketogenic diet, I am finding gluten and dairy free easy. The thing that I am most enjoying is eating whole grains and legumes again.

I am in awe with the confrontation of how much the perception of difficulty when it comes to food limits, just like everything else in life, is relative. Theoretically knowing something is not the same thing as living it, and I am glad for this experience.

Regarding how it feels to re-introduce carbs, I do have a slightly bloated stomach and a fair bit of gas, although I am eating very healthy whole foods. I had considered doing the paleolithic diet after the ketogenic, so as to re-introduce different macronutrients more gradually after a month of eating almost exclusively fat, but the thought of eating limited carbs for another entire month made me sad.

So suffer through this intestinal discomfort I must, and be patient as my digestion tract and all its components adjust.

Day 14

I can't believe two weeks have gone by without me having written about this food challenge. To be honest, although I have not cheated, it has not been easy to stay enthusiastic and faithful to no gluten and no dairy.

After the strict ketogenic diet, the problem is not that I don't have enough choices of what to eat, because in comparison, I do have many choices. The problem is that I am starting to tire of the food limits and simply want to eat whatever I want to eat.

This means that in order not to give up completely, I am back to frequently struggling with myself and fighting with my internal voices. When I am on the cusp of cheating, I start thinking to myself, "No one cares about your stupid food challenges," or "Why are you doing these dumb experiments?" It amazes me that it is the perception of how important or unimportant my actions are to others that come up as an excuse to cheat.

On the other hand, the motivation to not cheat brings up a completely opposite inner talk, which is directed within and in the vein of "Hang in there, you can do it!" or "you have come this far, don't stop now". I wonder if there is a lesson to be learnt from the clear discrepancy between the subjects of the externally versus internally oriented inner voices that can be applied to other parts of my life.

Regarding how I feel physically, the good news is that I feel great. I believe that I can get all the nutrients I need from the plethora of dairy and gluten free food choices. Furthermore, the consecutive and always changing food challenges have given me a huge amount of experience with different foods and cooking styles, so I feel completely happy spending time in the kitchen brewing up yummy dairy and gluten free stuff for me and the family to eat.

I also think I look well. Healthy, full of energy and in a positive mindset. Now I just have to get through this momentary lull in will power and hang in there... oh, there it is again, I recognize that internally oriented positive motivation inner talk.

Day 21

Today is Christmas day, and since my mom is getting divorced and moving to a more sustainable apartment, it was the last family holiday celebration at the big house.

I was afraid of the upcoming changes resulting in an overhanging negative or sad vibe, but everyone was in a great mood. We exchanged gifts, ate, drank wine, talked pleasantly, and were simply happy to be a family together.

Regarding the food challenges, although it was tough not to eat all the yummy cream based deserts typical of a Portuguese Christmas meal, the turkey, rich nutty rice, and chestnut stuffing were great. And so, of course, was the wine!

Day 30

And here it is, the end of this challenge and very little to say. Unlike all previous challenges, this was less of a food challenge than an experiment in will power. Even though there were always options when it came to food, after eight months into this project, I am feeling saturated of the food limitations.

The New Year holiday was especially difficult. Patrick and I spent a few days in a very fancy hotel/spa in

Algarve (Bela Vista, Portimão) where the most beautiful breads and cheeses were put out each morning for breakfast in a beautiful glass enclosed dining room surrounded by the ocean with its impressive rocky landscape. There were no gluten free starchy alternatives like oat or rice breads or crackers, so I had to satisfy myself with soft boiled eggs or eggs fried in olive oil and various wonderful types of fruit.

New Year's Eve dinner, which was celebrated with friends and their family, was also quite a challenge. Especially at desert time, where every amazing piece of cake or pudding was made with milk, cream and/or wheat flour. Although I still haven't done a month on the paleolithic diet (which I will hereafter interchangeably refer to as simply paleolithic or paleo), this challenge often felt similar to what paleo will be like.

As such, I feel that I ate a lot of animal protein, vegetables and fruits this past month. Regarding my weight, I weighed in at 58.7 kg this morning, which is 100 g more that on the first day of this challenge. This is a good result, considering that we had Christmas and New Year's holiday celebrations.

Conclusion

I don't have much to conclude about this month as far as food goes. However, even if it was easy to do in regard to cooking and eating, it was a tough game of personal will power and strength not to give up and eat whatever I wanted.

Unlike the last time I lived gluten free for 30 days, beer

was not an issue, and although I felt like a cold beer sometimes, it was easy to avoid. The thing I missed the most was cheese. I now realize how much I just love cheese. Today, on my day off, I immediately had some Dutch cheese accompanied by soft-boiled eggs for breakfast.

In general, I found this challenge to be similar to a paleolithic style diet, especially when eating out of the house, and I am curious to compare it to my upcoming paleo challenge in a few months.

Positives
- It was very difficult to find "permitted" processed foods, due to wheat, dairy or both being in the ingredient list of most junk food.
- Found this challenge not difficult to do after the keto challenge, although this is probably true for any diet that follows a strict ketogenic diet.
- I felt energic and slept well.
- I feel very proud of myself for having managed to hang in there and stay with it through the seasonal festivities.
- Maintained my weight without dieting at all.
- Experimented with different foods, like for example making excellent oatmeal with nuts, banana and vegetable milks as well as an excellent black rice and seafood dish.

Negatives
It was difficult to stay away from high quality cheeses and milky/creamy deserts, especially throughout the

holidays.
- I believe that my body needs milk products to feel completely healthy and am right now feeling that my joints are slightly fragile, although this may be because of age or because it's winter.
- I don't like limitations and am getting tired of not being able to eat whatever I feel like.

My day off
A dairy day from beginning to end. Cheese and eggs for breakfast, a Greek salad with Feta cheese for lunch, and a much-desired creamy pasta for dinner. Feeling good, and ready for one more dairy free month.

In retrospect
Looking back after going through all the food challenges, I feel the need to mention that these 30-days were followed by macrobiotic, paleo and vegan months. This means that this was the first dairy free month of four in a row. After basically going four months without dairy, and looking back over my complaints this month, I must clarify that my weakness in the joints did not persist and was therefore not due to lack of dairy.
Before I get into how important I think this month was in terms of how it solidified the process and allowed for the completion of this project. As I wrote somewhere in my entries during this experiment, I found this month to be more about gaining momentum to stay with the project than about the challenge itself.
I am not sure where my brain was at this point

regarding what I was expecting for the final outcome of these challenges to be. I don't remember if I had decided that I was going to write a book, but I think it was approximately during this time that the possibility of turning my logs into a book arose. Which brings me back to the significance of the process that allowed for the eventual completion of this project.

I have two close friends from my beach ultimate world (Pedro Vargas and Rui Pires)that I consider gurus and with whom I love to discuss performance and sport psychology. Pedro and Rui have been present throughout the entire challenges year, and I have thoroughly enjoyed talking to them both.

When I bounced the paragraph about inner talk and motivation with Pedro on messenger to see if it made sense, he replied – and resilience results from a balance between intrinsic and extrinsic motivation. This led to a whole conversation about the difference between being task (process) oriented or goal (outcome) oriented.

Using sports as an example, and simplifying things, an outcome oriented athlete works to win, whereas a task oriented athlete works to improve a specific task or to surpass a previously conquered milestone. For me, the completion of this month represents another task, or part of the process, that was successfully met. In the end, the eighth task of twelve which allowed me to reach the final goal of completing the year.

This book, as the outcome, was probably only considered to be a possibility at some point after successfully getting through this month. And this, was undoubtedly due to a lot of intrinsic (me) and extrinsic (my family and friends) motivation and support.

Gluten and dairy free revisited – November 2018

Reading over the in-retrospect section of this challenge, I am at a loss for words to add. Growth is multi processed, and objectives are important. But, showing up for the job and doing the boring stuff is part of it too... and doing it to the best of our abilities is tough. Especially when it gets tedious, boring, or repetitive.

Cooking for example, which I love, sometimes can be a royal pain in the butt. There are days that I just don't feel like even thinking about what to make, never mind putting my body into it. In those cases, if there is no other choice, I try to flip my mind around. I take a deep breath, start thinking about the ingredients in the house, and then focus on enjoying making a meal and hopefully sharing it with someone.

Like anything in life, it's best to not waste time fighting doing something that you simply must do. Ideally, harness the time spent doing whatever you have to do for mental relaxation, moments for conscious awareness, or for concentrating on something and letting go of all else.

chapter 9 - macrobiotic

For the ninth month of food experiments, I am going to eat guided by the macrobiotic principles for 30 days. There are many reasons that I chose to do this challenge, including that it used to be the food and lifestyle mode of the founder of the Institute for Integrative Nutrition, Joshua Rosenthal, who through the coaching program has greatly inspired me over the last few years to explore my own food self.

More great to try macrobiotic is that this eating style is highly flexible regarding what can be eaten. Moreover, it is a diet rich in whole grains, which I miss terribly after a keto month followed by a gluten free month. The origins of the macrobiotic diet are based on the ancient Japanese theory of yin and yang, with the general concept being that we should eat whole foods grown as locally and as organically as possible.

According to macrobiotic guidelines, whole grains make up most of what we should be eating (the base of the macrobiotic pyramid) and these should be complemented by plant foods such as beans, chickpeas, vegetables (excluding night shades such as tomatoes, peppers, asparagus, potatoes, eggplant and zucchini, which are to be avoided), fermented soybeans (such as soy sauce, tempeh, tofu, miso), some fruits (no tropical fruits), some seeds and nuts, seaweed and some fish.

Red meat, chicken, dairy, coffee, alcohol, and eggs are to be avoided, as is any processed food. The only thing that I am worried about is the no dairy limit, as I feel it is an important part of my diet. This "missing my dairy foods now and in anticipation" feeling is exacerbated by the fact that I still want to try paleo and vegan after this month, meaning that dairy based foods are going to be scarce for the rest of the experimental year.

Day 1

Today I opened the computer and googled "Macrobiotic" as a search term. After opening the "Macrobiotic Diet" article on Wikipedia*, I was taken aback to read in the conceptual paragraph, "Macrobiotics takes a view of health which contradicts science (Clow B, 2001)".

Thinking further about this statement and taking into account that the origin of macrobiotic dates back to 1797 Japan, this is actually not surprising. Not only has the way we eat greatly changed in the last two hundred years, there have been significant advances in our knowledge of nutrition and dietary science.

Also, like for many other "diet lifestyle/theories", it is important not to lose the context around the birth of the theory. The macrobiotic diet originated and initially developed in one geographical location and therefore designed to meet the needs and provide guidelines adjusted to that specific reality.

The health benefits of eating locally, or more specifically, plants that are growing around you, is a very valid point. However, it is just as important to realize that different things grow in different places around the world. I believe it is essential to consider cultural/geographical differences. For example, one guideline in macrobiotic is to avoid tropical fruits. As much sense as this makes if you want to eat fresh plant foods in Japan, why should these foods be avoided if you live in the tropics?

The one thing I find highly positive about this diet/lifestyle is that it is based on guidelines rather than absolutes. For instance, in the case of red meat, the macrobiotic approach would state that it should be avoided most of the time, rather than forbidding that red meat be eaten.

Regardless of the merits and fails of this diet/lifestyle, there are some things that completely resonate with me and my philosophy surrounding food and the ritual of eating. I do think it is important to be grateful for each meal, as well believe in the benefits of chewing every bite carefully. Although 50 chews may be an exaggeration, we do eat too quickly. Slowing down, chewing properly, and enjoying our meals is important for our digestive and nervous systems.

So far, I am enjoying and looking forward to this experiment. I am also happy to be going to the Instituto Macrobiótico de Portugal (Portuguese Macrobiotic Institute) with my friend Noélia next Tuesday to learn more.

On a fun note, today I made my first miso soup for lunch, with seaweed, bock choy and tofu. I loved it, although I did get complaints from the rest of the family that the house smelt like fish sauce. Also, I have already placed dried chickpeas in water to hydrate overnight and to use for cooking tomorrow.

Day 3

I feel like am gently rolling into the macrobiotic mind frame and am thoroughly enjoying the journey. It feels very alike to a warm hug on a cold day. Lucky that I picked this time of year, the dead of winter, for this experiment. I am loving cooking as well as eating whole grains, softly and slowly cooked vegetables, legumes, and sometimes fish, slightly spiced with soy, salt, miso or seaweed.

One thing is for sure, I am thoroughly enjoying learning about the macrobiotic cookware and cooking styles. It has been great fun learning and using new cooking methods and ingredients. Yesterday I bought organic whole grain rice syrup. What a great natural sweetener, cheap and due to its lack of strong taste, very versatile!

Day 8

This week, I had the pleasure of going for lunch with a long-term scientist friend, Noélia Custódio, who knows a lot about macrobiotic and loosely follows a macrobiotic lifestyle. Our outing felt like a research fieldtrip, and I learnt a lot from her extensive macrobiotic schooling.

We met and had lunch at the Portuguese Macrobiotic Institute, which is in a beautifully renovated old building in downtown Lisbon. I love the feel of the place; the food is always great, and the environment is cozy and warm.

There is a small macrobiotic small shop at the Institute,

with books and other educational material. And foods, so I bought some barley Miso and my friend offered me some seaweed and sesame salt to welcome me into this new experiment.

In general, I am thoroughly enjoying this challenge and notice that it is triggering some significant changes in my food self, and not just cooking and eating. For one thing, I am chewing much more frequently per bite, which means that I eat much slower and am often the last one at the table with food on my plate. Also, I am in a very positive mind-frame even though I haven't been sleeping great the last week (too many monkeys making noise and playing around in my brain).

I do feel that this is the perfect time for macrobiotic, not only because it is winter but also there are no frisbee tournaments or anything else that I need to be physically competitive for. In general, this diet makes me feel soft and warm and lovey. I do miss meat and cheese, but I know it's only for a relatively short time, so its ok.

Day 15

Half way through the macrobiotic challenge and I am now at the point that I miss eating meat, eggs, chicken, and milk products. Also, I find it frustrating to have to avoid sweet potatoes (yams), zucchinis, and avocados, which are normally a regular part of my diet.

On a positive note, I do enjoy the whole grains and love to incorporate miso in my vegetable stews. Also, I like that there is some flexibility in macrobiotics for a little wine, beer, and some sweets such as softly baked apple crumble.

Day 25

I can't believe that there are only five days to go until the end of the ninth month of challenges. Although I am still enjoying this regime, I am very much looking forward to the next challenge, which will be almost the polar-opposite approach to eating – the paleolithic diet! But for now, off to cook more grains.

Day 30

Oh, I am happy that today is the end day and can't wait to bite into some eggs and meats. Also, I seriously plan to load up on dairy on my day off, since dairy has been off-limits the last two months and will continue to be so for the next few challenges. My husband Patrick went to Holland a couple of weeks ago and brought back some wonderful cheeses that are patiently waiting in the fridge for me. I guess that for the next few challenges days off will be dairy days!

Conclusion

What a wonderful experience this month was. I loved learning about macrobiotic, and mostly found the foods and lifestyle guidelines to be a very pleasant experience. Especially during these cold and rainy winter months.

I do think that it helped that I was going through a non-physically demanding phase of the year, without any competitive events and without any demanding muscle stimulation/strength training. I think this curbed my instinctual need for meat protein.

I did enjoy fish on average twice a week. Interestingly, I found there to be some similarities and overlaps between Portuguese food and macrobiotic, especially the legume dishes such as bean stew and chick-pea dishes, as well the potted fish and rice dishes or vegetable stews.

Regarding my weight, I did lose 1.4 kg this month, weighing in at 57.3 kg this morning. This is less than at the end of the keto month although my waist circumference is the same as it was then, measuring in at 82 cm.

Overall, although I enjoyed macrobiotic, I am getting tired of having food limitations of any kind. Nine months is a long time, enough time to make a human baby. On the other hand, somehow the limits have opened new paths, and I have learnt a load about cultures, foods, and myself in this process.

Positives
- Enjoyed incorporating macrobiotic spices (or non-spices that add flavor) into my cooking, especially miso, seaweed, and sea salted sesame seeds.
- Once again, it was a pleasure finding alternatives to satisfy my sweet tooth. One great new sweetener that we are all happy for the discovery of is rice jelly. It is affordable, and if I am a firm believer that if we eat something sweet, it is advisable to vary the sources by using various dark sugars, honey, maple syrup, etcetera. After

this month, rice jelly will surely become a regular in my pantry. Very good indeed.

- Felt great energy, slept well and maintained regular intestinal health throughout the month.
- Lost a bit of weight without any effort, which may be due to muscle loss because of the lull in serious training lately… but I feel good and feel that I look good.
- I really enjoyed some of the macrobiotic inspired "behavioral adaptations" around food, such as consciously appreciating the meal at hand. And practicing mindful eating, including trying to chew 50 times per bite. Probably closer to 20 or 30 for me, but I did notice changes.
- Loved eating grains again, which I really missed after the last challenge and will likely miss terribly in the upcoming paleo month.
- Very interesting to see that although my diet was 60 % grains, I did not have any intestinal issues.

Negatives
- As in previous dairy-free months, it was very difficult to stay away from high quality cheeses and yogurts. This is especially complicated for me because I believe milk products are an integral part of my diet. Dutch cheese and yogurt are still a part of our household and my family's diet, I just can't eat either. Unlike the previous month, my joints felt ok without dairy, perhaps because I have not been training intensively this month.

- Besides the fact that I don't like limitations, I found some of the theories of macrobiotic dubious at best. Mostly because its origin is that of a whole food diet in Japan in the late 1700s, and therefore it is not applicable to all places. For example, why could I not eat avocados or sweet potatoes when they grow just outside my house? Sometimes I found this diet to be a bit silly and not necessarily health promoting. But this, I believe, is usually the case when any feeding limitation is imposed by what we hold as being the truth and are too rigid to forget to apply it to the moment at hand. Food limitations should be based on respect for our bodies, exploring new foods, and learning how we react to certain foods.

My day off

Once again, I overdid it on dairy, especially knowing that there are another two "dairy free" challenges coming up. It felt great to eat whatever I wanted, especially cheese and meat!

In retrospect

Reading over this month, I had forgotten how much I enjoyed macrobiotic and the large influence this challenge had on the types of ingredients readily available in the house.

It was very nice to have an old science friend, Noélia, to teach me about the basic concepts of this diet/lifestyle and to accompany me on a field trip to the Portuguese Macrobiotic Institute, a place that I very much like.

With all this talk about macrobiotic foods and since I hadn't had lunch yet, I was immediately inspired to make a "macrobiotic-fusion-style" hummus, with sesame, organic sea salt, barley miso, olive oil, softly roasted garlic, and chickpeas. I am enjoying it right now over a bed of salad and wondering why this month was so easy... drifted by... came and went without any major bumps, slumps, or moments of desperation.

I guess that is why it didn't leave a strong impression on me. I'm glad I got the opportunity to edit and re-live it, as it brought a pleasant experience that had been archived somewhere in the attic of my brain to the fore-front of my mind.

Macrobiotic revisited – November 2018

I personally learned some invaluable lessons from this month, especially around the act of eating. In the current times, we often forget where food comes from... never mind thanking the universe for the opportunity to eat it. And the act of eating itself, a slow and peaceful process where every bite is made conscious. What a concept for the busy folk on this planet, who tend to eat food quickly so can go do whatever needs to get done!

Regarding the macrobiotic lifestyle, I believe that there are many changes going on regarding how the theory is developing. As is the case for any theory, different schools arise from the interpretation of the changing science and its fit into the existing dogma.

Regardless of the food guidelines of macrobiotic, I do appreciate the lack of severity, it shows a respect for human individuality. My lesson was that making time for food is what counts.

I try to coach my clients to guarantee that at least one meal a day is home cooked, and that it is enjoyed sitting down at a table (or around in a circle). Sometimes travel and busy lives make us lose perspective of the basics, like food. But eating high quality foods with a positive mindset is health promoting from every aspect!

References

From Wikipedia*: Clow B (2001). *Negotiating Disease: Power and Cancer Care, 1900-1950*. McGill-Queen's University Press. p. 63. Before we explore medical reactions to therapeutic innovations in this era, we must stop to consider the meaning of 'alternative medicine' in this context. Often scholars use the term to denote systems of healing that are philosophically as well as therapeutically distinct from regular medicine: homeopathy, reflexology, rolfing, macrobiotics, and spiritual healing, to name a few, embody interpretations of health, illness, and healing that are not only different from, but also at odds with conventional medical opinion.

*This reference was cited in a log entry dated January 5, 2017. The Wikipedia article for "Macrobiotic Diet" has since been altered and the conceptual basis no longer contains this reference nor the statement that the macrobiotic diet contradicts science. (June 28, 2017)

Chapter 10 – paleolithic diet

The tenth challenge and the one that I have been most curious about is finally here, the paleolithic diet (hereafter also referred to as paleo)! There is an image forever engraved in my mind's eye associated with the first time I heard of this diet, which was during the health coach training program at the Institute for Integrative Nutrition.

The lecturer, a strong advocate of the paleo diet/lifestyle, was a testosterone empowered man dressed in a tight black t-shirt and jeans, with a faux-hawk and lots of protruding muscles. Whilst walking around on stage like a caged large feline and talking about how we have lost our full potential as humans, he showed an image to make his point. This image - which did I mention I will never forget? - was of a chihuahua dog and a wolf.

According to paleo, our current eating habits are not potentiating our best selves, and the contrasting image of the wolf and the chihuahua was to show our transformation from our "full potential selves" into the modern-day man. To be our best, we should be eating more like hunters and gatherers. I loved the dramatic effect of his delivery, his male strength, and even some of the theory.

The paleolithic diet is very rich in theory, so please bear with me as I go into it before diving into my cave-woman experience. Again, skip it if you wish, although I really hope you don't.

The Paleolithic period extends from the earliest known use of stone tools by our ancestors, circa 2.6 million years ago, to approximately 10 000 before the present time. It was during the Paleolithic era that the anatomically and behaviorally "modern" human is believed to have emerged in eastern Africa at least 200 000 years before the present time.

It is thought that by around 50 000 before present, we started expanding throughout the planet. Initially making it to Europe and Australia, followed by Japan, Siberia and eventually to the Arctic Circle. By the end of the Paleolithic, humans had crossed from what is today modern Russia to modern Canada and quickly expanded throughout the Americas.

Our gradual evolution from early members of the genus *Homo* into modern and much larger brained humans (*Homo sapiens sapiens*) was likely intimately associated with our dispersal. We are an extremely adaptable species. This is especially true when it comes to how we get adequate nutrients for proper functioning.

Nearly all of our knowledge of Paleolithic human culture and way of life comes from studies of modern tribal cultures who live as contemporary hunter-gatherers, similarly to their Paleolithic predecessors. As far as we know, humans grouped together in small societies consisting of less than 100 individuals, and subsisted by gathering plants, fishing, hunting or scavenging wild animals.

One interesting aspect of the hunter-gatherer lifestyle that drastically changed in future Neolithic farming societies and modern industrial societies is that

Paleolithic humans enjoyed an abundance of leisure time. As a small aside, I have to admit that I like this fact and believe boredom often empowers creativity and ingenuity. I would dare to say that boredom has become a luxury in the digital age, where there is a tendency to pick up the phone, go on the computer, or watch a screen of some kind when bored. The brain goes to somewhere around zero, you may still be bored, but it is not likely to be very productive.

A little boredom is health promoting as well as allows for great creative thoughts. Especially in children, who will come up with the coolest things to do when bored. Bored comments aside, let's get back to the paleo diet.

My highly critical scientific mind has a tough time swallowing the concept of a diet/lifestyle based on a period of human history encompassing more than 2 million years. Add to that a geographical area covering most of our planet. Defining a diet for this era seems impossible. We populated many habitats as hunters and gatherers, and thrived on various diets.

Consider how much has changed in how we eat over the last 150 years and the cultural differences that exist between our food ingredients and cooking styles across continents today. And this in a global society, where information exchange can travel over large geographical regions in merely seconds.

Not to add more entropy to the paleo dietary concept, but there were also significant geographic and climatic changes during the Paleolithic era (Pleistocene epoch of geologic time) which had large effects on prehuman and human societies. Obviously, this had a huge influence on their food and feeding.

The paleo diet/lifestyle supports the theory that not enough time has passed for our biological systems to have evolved to deal with foods products from agriculture, which started at least 10 000 years ago. Therefore, according to the paleo theory, foods from crops such as grains and dairy from domesticated animals are highly detrimental to our health.

What I find particularly interesting, and this is a small scientific aside, is the comparatively recent evolution of the B antigen in human blood, which is present in people with blood types B or AB. The B blood antigen is believed to have initially appeared between 10,000 and 15 000 years ago in the Himalayan highlands. Since the B blood antigen has been estimated to have initially appeared at the time when farming started, it is often associated with dairy tolerance.

There is one more thing I think is important to note, on my thread to refute strict paleo. The significant increase in brain size we underwent during the paleolithic era was undoubtably related to our increased exposure to variable environments. Just think about the increase in mobility and therefore augmented exposure to different environments, foods, shelters, social systems and so on that occurred when we came out of the trees.

There are likely many factors that influenced our evolution. Food? Yes, we ate what we could. We are a highly resilient species when it comes to nutrition, and can assimilate macro-nutrients from many sources. A fact that no doubt influenced our dispersal. As of course did agriculture, allowing for populations to stay in one place permanently and build farming communities.

Ok, now that some of the science as well as my doubts and criticisms of the theoretical basis behind this eating style are out of the way, let us go along with the premise that we can define a paleo "hunter and gatherer" diet. I don't see myself eating grubs or chunks of meat straight from the still-warm carcass, so I will assume this diet as a modern version of what was consumed when our brains went through their greatest expansion. That's what this month will be about, the "modern paleo" diet.

Since I cannot eat foods from agriculture, that means that grains or sugars are off limits, although I would bet you that any caveman gorged on all the ripe fruit or honey combs that he/she came across. But I do believe that sugars are a drug, at least for most of the population, and that there would be much less inflammation and auto-immune disease in our population if they were used as such.

Regarding what I am allowed to eat on the paleo diet, there is some controversy regarding consumption of dairy, and so I intend to follow a strict version of no dairy except for clarified butter that has no lactose and is highly similar to meat fat in nutritional content. Of course, processed foods are not allowed.

Considering that I cannot eat grains or legumes, this diet is basically the polar opposite of macrobiotic. I will be eating organic meats and fish, nuts, all veggies (except potato), low glycemic index fruits, and eggs.

As a diet/lifestyle, the paleo diet is very popular right now. I think I can safely venture to say that with paleo cook books, ingredients, courses, sports bars, etcetera, it is a multimillion dollar industry. Athletes love it as the high protein content in this diet is ideal for muscle synthesis and therefore aids in getting "pumped". Housewives love it because it is great for thinning out.

Personally, I am looking forward to this month. To add incentive to this challenge, I have joined the gym and intend to hit the weight room hard. As a cavewoman at the gym, I hope to increase my lean body mass and shed a little more body fat, which will hopefully result in better explosive performance playing disc.

Day 1

One day into my cave-woman month and I am already missing grains and dairy. This is not going to be easy. On the other hand, I do get to eat all kinds of yummy things that I like (it's a good thing that I am an optimist). Speaking of good foods and cooking ideas, I went online to look for what I paleo foods that I may like to make and eat.

While searching google for recipes on Pinterest using "paleo" and "recipes" as search terms, I was flabbergasted by the incredibly high number of results. Considering that it is supposedly a caveman diet, I found it amusing to see that most of paleo recipes were highly elaborate and appetizing.

Also very funny, there were loads of recipes for "paleo breads, cakes and muffins", which in itself is contradictory considering that baked goods were invented as a way to eat grains from crops (breads were made from fermented grain flour).

Anyway, I look at the amazing fancy images of paleo cooking and it makes me laugh to imagine caveman internet and fancy cooking machines like blenders, juicers and ovens. In a way it's good news for me, considering that raw meat and raw nuts are just not that appetizing.

Day 3

I have never eaten so much meat in my life, I almost feel like growling! Seriously, although I thoroughly enjoy meat, fish and nuts, this diet has too much animal protein for me. Also, even though I eat whenever I'm hungry, I miss the complex starchy carbs and legumes to the point that I often feel unsatisfied.

I have noticed is that this diet is very expensive. This is especially true because it is important for me to eat high quality meats and fish, which means that I only buy organic meats and wild salmon. Taken together with the nuts and berries, this is not a diet for the economically challenged.

Regarding fitness, I have joined a gym close by with Patrick and my daughter Sara. After my evaluation at the gym this week, I made a conscious decision to reduce my body fat and increase muscle mass. I really believe paleo will help.

In a way, this eating regime reminds me of the ketogenic diet from a few months ago, although without the high fat dairy and allowing for a lot more fruits and vegetables. Although I do miss my grains and dairy, I am nowhere near to cheating.

Day 7

After one week as a cave woman and I am rocking paleo! Of course, nothing is mono-factorial, and I am sure that part of the reason I feel like I do is because I joined the gym and am regularly exercising in the weight room as well as playing or practicing disc at least twice a week.

Day 12

Besides the fact that it is extremely difficult not to dig my teeth into the freshly baked bread that is staring at me every morning at the local bakery, I am still enjoying paleo. In fact, much more than I thought I would.

During the first week, I missed starches and often felt that although I was not necessarily hungry after a meal, something was missing. Gladly, I have found ways around this by baking paleo friendly pancakes, tortillas, and even cakes made from bananas, eggs, coconut oil (or olive oil) and then various seeds and nuts pulverized (or not) into flour. Very good indeed!

I am actually enjoying this so much, and feel so good, that I am starting to dread the idea of trying vegan next month. Hmmm, I am having a ha-ha moment, maybe I will go vegan-paleo... that will definitely get the extra fat off my stomach area.

Day 22

I am still thoroughly enjoying being a cave-woman.

And even though it is not easy to stay away from starches or legumes, I feel great and powerful. Funny that I also think that this diet is influencing my behavior by specifically increasing my directness. In fact, sometimes I'm surprised about what comes out of my mouth and almost want to look back and see who just said that (me?).

I also notice that this eating regime is affecting my entire family immensely. My husband, who is an avid meat lover, has been enjoying going out of his way to make great paleo meals. We also bought a small "veggie peeler" that can cut vegetables into spaghetti like strings, which is fantastic for making zucchini noodles (zoodles).

I can't believe that there is only one more week to go – I am not looking forward to the next and second-last challenge. But until then, I still have a beach ultimate tournament to play as a cave-woman. Curious to see how playing seven games over two days without any simple carbs between matches goes.

Day 30

Playing a tournament on a strict Paleo diet was not easy. I felt great going into the tournament, full of energy, strong and in shape... the problem was later in the day.

Considering my team was the organizational team and therefore had to set up fields, tents, and all other sorts of organizational activities as well as play, the weekend was very physically challenging. I founds that it was impossible for me to maintain the same amount of energy for four games in a row without eating some quick digestion starchy carbs. I didn't, but felt increasingly tired as the day went on.

On the night after the first day, and after a complete Paleo dinner of meats and fruits, I felt very sleepy and in need of something else to eat. Thank goodness, I got into the people and the party and continued on my dancing paleo way. By bedtime, I was thoroughly happy with the day and internally laughing while re-living the random moments that you often experience with the frisbee crowd.

Luckily for me, the challenge ended on the first day of the tournament and the second day was my day off, which means that I could eat anything. And, better yet, drink beer with my team after the games were over.

Conclusion

I was surprised what a great month it was eating like a modern hunter and gatherer cave-woman. I did not expect to enjoy eating so much animal protein, which was truly a pleasure!

In a sense, I have to laugh when I think of the fancy amazing paleo recipes that both Patrick and I concocted this month, nothing "cavey" about these meals. Also, I tend to eat slowly and chew a lot lately, also not an eating behavior I visualize as being how our ancestors ate.

The modern paleo is all about adapting to the modern world, and this diet/lifestyle has adapted quite well to the western society's current need to cut down on pro-inflammatory foods. As I mentioned before and think is important to note, although the quality of foods that the paleo diet supports is excellent, with all its nuts and meats, this regime is not light on the wallet. Also, it is not a diet that is light on the planet.

As far as the environmental footprint, our current meat industry places a heavy load on our environment. We should be eating more plants, and we should be able to take advantage of the great healthy gains that we can get from grains and legumes. Ha-ha, that is a great saying! Great gains from grains…Try to say that three times in a row without screwing up!

Regarding my physical self, I felt great during this paleo month. I had plenty of energy and strength for my active daily life, including training, working, and enjoying my family. Regarding the effects of the paleo diet on athletic capacity, in an interesting review of the merits of popular diets on weight loss and athletic performance.

The author, Rosenbloom (2014), clarifies the importance for athletes to recognize the limitations inherent to specific diets and work with a sports dietitian to modify feeding plans to meet their unique needs. Although all weight-loss diets work in the short term, there do not appear to be long-term benefits of any of these, including paleo, on athletic performance.

In this vein, although I was strong and feeing fit all month at the gym and playing disc, I was exhausted by the end of the first day of the two-day beach ultimate tournament. I think quick digesting carbs would have helped. Regarding body parameters, I thinned out a bit this month, and now weigh in at 56.7 kg and have a waist circumference of 78 cm. That is a 600 g weight loss and a 4 cm loss in waist circumference. Of course, these results are likely influenced by the regularity of my physical activity, which include regular sessions of strength training at the gym (four times per week) and disc (at least two times per week).

Positives
- Surprisingly, I thoroughly enjoyed eating so much meat, fish, and eggs.
- As with all previous challenges, it was a pleasure to find alternatives for my sugar cravings and to became an expert at making sweet potato pancakes and cookies.
- Just like with most challenges, I felt great energy, slept well and my intestines were amazingly regular. In fact, I did notice a difference in the quickness and regularity of bowel movements. Paleo power dumps!
- Felt fantastic at the gym and that my body responded well to physical strength and conditioning training. Also, and probably related, I lost 600 g and 4 cm waist circumference. In general, I feel like my body is getting where I want it to be... I feel increasingly good and feel that I look good.
- Very interesting to see that I can live without the products of agriculture. Considering how difficult my initial gluten free month was, I am pleasantly surprised at how much easier this month was,

even though I could not eat rice or any other grain.
- It was very difficult to find unhealthy food choices with paleo.
- All in all, this challenge was an unexpected wonderful experience.

Negatives
- As with all the other challenges that exclude dairy foods, it was very difficult to stay away from high quality cheeses and yogurts. On the other hand, I must emphasize that even though I have been doing regular strength and disc training, I did not have pain in my joints without dairy.
- Also, and a recurring theme when it comes to food regimes, I found some of the theories behind paleo comical at best. Especially when I think of the fancy recipes that were served up to my family this month.
- Paleo is expensive.

My day off
Wow, I ate a load of cheese on my day off! And beer! It was oh-so-good to bite into the dry bits and corners of wonderful Dutch cheeses that had been waiting in the fridge for me to be out of the paleo month. And beer, oh boy did beer taste good! Oh so good!
I spent my whole day off playing beach ultimate at a tournament, organizing, drinking beer, and eating anything I felt like (bread with Nutella tasted awesome). Since it was the second and final day of the

tournament, which is hosted by our team, we finished off the day at a restaurant celebrating.

The tournament is called Lisbon MOW, and is fantastic thanks to the impressive and highly positive organization from three frisbee buddies, including Carla and Dani who are also teammates and great friends. Way to end my cave-woman month... eating pizza and cheesecake accompanied by sweet Lambrusco wine with the team. OMG, that was awesome!

In retrospect

Before I get into the highly positive aspects of the paleolithic diet, bear with me as I lay one more recent scientific finding on you that I immediately found relevant while reading it a couple of weeks ago. Ancient stone tools dating back to 3.3 million years, which is pre-paleolithic, were recently found in Kenya.

This shows that we started using tools much earlier than previously thought. Also, it puts previously calculated chronological estimates of when our brains started expanding in question. It may have occurred earlier than previously thought.

Regardless of the flaws in the whole concept of being able to define a diet that encompasses over 2 million years and the entire planet, our modern concept of paleo was a pleasure to do. I was not expecting to enjoy this month half as much as I did. I felt great, loved the foods, and was completely surprised by Patrick's coming on board and loving being a cave-man too. At least at dinner time, when he made the most amazing and tasty meals, including the now family favored noodles from zucchini (zoodles).

Regarding our health, there are huge advantages to paleo, mostly because agriculture is banned and therefore processed foods are out. Did it have a long-term effect on the way we and I eat? Yes. Whether by itself or in combination with the ketogenic and gluten free challenges, it definitely did! I eat paleo meals often nowadays. Also, I no longer consider the need for starchy accompaniments such as bread, rice, potatoes, or pasta in my meals.

Tonight, Patrick made a fantastic zoodle dish with shrimp and a lime-coconut creamy sauce for dinner. Another big change is that I eat eggs much more often than I used to, and eggs with many vegetables is a oftentimes a family breakfast or lunch favorite. Taken together, this means that there are noticeable differences in how long bread lasts in our household in comparison to what it used to last.

Paleolithic revisited – November 2018

The most solid knowledge that we get from nutrition science is that our bodies are extremely resilient and adaptable to different foods. Our capacity to utilize calories from different sources of foods makes us adaptable to various environments, which partially explains our quick spread throughout the globe.

An interesting discovery has been recently published regarding our origins (Sprinter 2016). Morphologic and genetic results from fossil records show that our last common ancestor from the Neanderthals, our closest cousins, was between 400 000 and 700 000 years ago.

This may indicate that our species arose at least 200 000 years earlier than previously thought.

References

Rosenbloom C. 2014. Popular Diets and Athletes Premises, Promises, Pros, and Pitfalls of Diets and What Athletes Should Know About Diets and Sports Performance, Nutrition Today, Vol. 49, pp. 244

Stringer C1. 2016. The origin and evolution of Homo sapiens. Philos Trans R Soc Lond B Biol Sci. Vol. 5;371 pp. 1698

Wong K. 2017. The new origins of technology. Scientific American, Vol. 316, pp. 22

Chapter 11 – vegan

Here we are on the second-last and much dreaded eleventh month of 30-day food challenges, no animal products. I never thought I would be able to go vegan, and to be honest, I am slightly reluctant... especially after enjoying being a cave woman for a month. On the other hand, I have gained a load of experience cooking and eating animal food alternatives this year and am looking forward to the challenge.

There are many who strongly advocate the health benefits of a vegan diet, and if you are interested in learning more about this I would suggest reading the book *The China Study* by T. Colin Campbell and Thomas M. Campbell and/or taking a look at https://www.forksoverknives.com.

There is no doubt that our footprint on the planet would be much less damaging if we all consumed a vegetable based diet. Just think of the huge number of calories of plant material necessary to feed a cow. Also, our current animal rearing practices are mostly focused on high production rather than quality.

Ideally, our meat should be coming from animals that are grazing in the fields. These are eating their natural food as well as returning nutrients back into the ground through their feces - valuable crop plant fertilizer. However, most of our meats come from animals which have been fed grain based feed, which is not their natural food. This results in high levels of inflammation and affects the quality of meat.

The quality of the meat is also influenced by extensive use of hormones and antibiotics in agribusiness. Besides that, the animal farming industry is conducive to a lot of food product waste at many levels along the production to consumption chain. Think of how much is wasted from live animal, to the store, to the kitchen, then the table and our guts.

Regardless of the many merits of a vegan diet for our planet, this month represents the first of the twelve challenges that imposes some nutrient deficiency issues. It lacks vitamin B12, which we can only bio-assimilate from animal based foods. Considering that we can store vitamin B12 in our livers for years, I will try not to supplement for the next month. Also, I am slightly worried about the decrease in healthy fish fats that I will be eating (EPA and DHA Omega 3) and wonder how that will affect my eyesight, especially at nightly practices on a somewhat lit beach. Of course, there is plenty of Omega 3 in plants, but not the longer carbon chained EPA and DHA, which I normally get a plenty of from my frequent sea food meals.

Day 1

Initiated my vegan month with a fantastic breakfast consisting of oatmeal made with almond milk and topped with loads of cinnamon, fruits, and nuts. Tasted great! I also started soaking some beans to make a rich bean soup.

I am curious about how much I will miss meats and fish and am going to try not to eat too much grains this month. Today, I am still physically exhausted from the tournament, but tomorrow I hope to hit the gym and see how I feel.

Day 2

Only two days have gone by and I am already hating the limitations imposed by this regime, especially when eating out. Yesterday was a friend's birthday and all I could eat at her party was chips and breadsticks, having to forego wonderful octopus and shrimp dishes as well as a fresh mushroom quiche and amazing cheeses.

Today I feel bloated and low in energy. On the positive side, I went shopping this morning for fresh greens and filled up a large bag with wonderful food for merely 7 Euros. This would be an impossible feat on the paleo diet.

Day 4

Feeling slightly gassy and bloated on day four as a vegan forager. Over the past two days, I have been eating a lot of healthy greens and legumes and avoiding breads and flour in general. I think my microbiome is going through a roller coaster ride and may take a while to adjust to the radical change in diet. Let's see how I feel in two weeks.

This month, there are a lot of close friend and family birthday celebrations, which can be socially difficult as a vegan. Yesterday, I took a friend's suggestion and ate dinner at home before going to a family dinner party (thanks Chris!). It was an interesting social experience to hang out at the party, enjoying chatting and eating salad. It was thought-provoking that no one noticed that there was anything different or odd about my eating, or lack of eating. The fact that I had already eaten dinner helped me not feel frustrated because of not being able to enjoy all the great foods being served.

Day 10

More than a week has gone by and I am drifting along into vegan much less painfully than I expected. No doubt that I thoroughly miss animal protein, especially eggs, meat and fish, but I also feel that there are enough options for me to make yummy meals at any time of day.

Today, at the suggestion of my health coach, I made a great and very simple tofu and coriander paste. Excellent to use on toast, salads, sautéed vegies, and so on. Simply blend tofu, salt, pepper and fresh coriander in the food processor to the consistency of a cream cheese. I personally like it sprinkled with a little olive oil and paprika.

There are more good news today in regards to this vegan experiment. My energy levels are great and after one week of adjusting, and my stomach/intestines are no longer rebelling against the diet changes incurred by the challenges.

It is strange to think that in a month and a half this whole year of experiments will be finished. That will be odd. Although it is highly likely that I will be repeating certain regimes as well as doing food experimentations and trying new food challenges for the rest of my life.

Day 11

I just arrived home from my book-club dinner and am seriously feeling the effects of my food limitations as I write this with a slight buzz. Dinner was interesting... another amazing night of highly intelligent complex women, not enough food, and a lot of great wine.

Our book club dinners are held in a wonderful second-hand book shop called *Dejá Lu*. I was informed that the restaurant had been warned that there would be one "nutritionally challenged" woman (me) who did not eat animal based foods.

When my beautiful dinner was placed in front of me, I immediately felt my head heat up in embarrassment. Staring at me and daring me to bite into it was a beautiful spinach and ricotta ravioli dish with cream sauce. Vegan? I don't think so.

Oh well, wine is vegan. In the end, everyone else enjoyed digging into my meal while I explained to the waiter and apologized for my limitations and asked for a salad. All's well that ends well, and once again I end up feeling a bit drunk after two or three glasses of white wine and very little food.

Day 21

Three weeks as a vegan and I have had enough of being a herbivore. Funny that after 4 months without eating dairy, I am not missing cheese or yogurt anymore. What I miss the most is eggs. and I can't wait to make myself a yum omelet!

On the other hand, I have been eating great vegan food.

Three days ago, I went with my health coach for lunch at a new place recently opened in Lisbon by a fellow health coach from the Institute for Integrative Nutrition, *Ohana by Naz*. Wonderful middle-eastern inspired food! I just loved eating various vegan dishes and desserts.

The thing about vegan that I find most tiring is that vegan dishes often need to be fairly elaborated to taste good to me. Thankfully, I like spending time cooking and have a pantry and fridge full of tasty ingredients to play with.

Another irritating aspect about this challenge, which is also shared by some other self-imposed food limitations I have tried this past year, is that vegan often forces me to make non-healthy food options. Just consider it: alcohol, sugar and chips are all vegan oks. Oh well. In general I do feel good, have been working out regularly, and am energetic and strong.

Day 28

Oh boy, I feel like absolute crap today. Funny to see how good and strong I was seven days ago, and now, exactly one week later, I am feeling physically weak, mentally grey, uninspired, and emotionally fragile.

Partially I think I am physically unwell, evident as a runny nose as well as an irritating scratchy cough. But also, and maybe not completely disconnected, this last week was the bearer of some disturbing news. We have just learnt of a close friend's potentially serious health issue while worrying about the impending lack of sufficient income to meet our family needs in the face of our quickly dwindling savings.

Generally, I tend not to worry or even think too much about money. Reflecting on why this is, I am not sure if it is because I am naturally irresponsible, if it is my upbringing (money was a taboo subject when I grew up), or just my inherent optimism. The simple truth is that I intrinsically believe things will work out financially. But not right now.

For some reason, Patrick's and my lack of regular income is making me anxious, heavy chested, and in a bad mood. I looked in the mirror today and I don't look very good. My husband thinks that the vegan diet is not helping my overall health, and I agree. But it is almost over. And to be honest, although I don't think I would ever choose to be a strict vegan, these last four weeks have not been as difficult as I was expecting.

Day 29

I am feeling much better today, and getting over my flu, body aches, sadness, and so on. Worked out hard again as well, and it was great to feel decently strong. Which brings me to the conclusion that although I still believe that I need animal protein, it wouldn't be fair to blame this diet regime for my down days.

Then again, I can't wait until it's over. I miss fish, eggs, and good old-fashioned butter immensely at this point. In fact, it makes me smile and drool just to think about how I am going to break my vegan diet with an awesome cheese and mushroom omelet for breakfast the day after tomorrow.

Day 30

Last day! Woohoo! Started off the day enjoying a couple of slices of seed and multigrain dark bread spread with tofu "cream cheese" accompanied by a green tea. Although it tasted great, the thought of the large and greasy cheese omelet that I will eat tomorrow morning did cross my mind while eating.

Vegan 30 days, I can't believe I did it! I had originally considered taking vitamin B12 supplements and Omega 3 from fish or algae (EPA and DHA), but did not feel the need. Which means that for the last 30 days, I managed to ingest exclusively plant foods and nutrients. Entirely plant based prime material for longer than the cycle of many of our cells. Wow! Am I glad that it is almost over? Yes!

Conclusion

Oh boy, I am so proud to have gotten through this one. Never in a million years did I think I could do it! I did learn a lot of new recipes (with tofu and seitan) and so did my husband.

I also lost some weight, which is surprising considering that I never went hungry except for the few times that I had dinner out and there were no vegan options. As far as metrics go, considering that this morning I weighed in at 55.7 kg and measured 77 cm around the waist, I lost 1 kg and 1 cm waist perimeter in the last month.

Did I like this diet? I must admit that no, I did not. I found that I often had to make the unhealthy choice when eating out to stay within plant foods. Also, I missed some favorites badly, such as eggs and fish.

It was interesting that cheese and milk products have somehow ceased to become a part of my cravings. I guess that after four consecutive dairy free months, these foods are no longer a conscious option when I am hungry. In the end, vegan was not as difficult as I thought it would be and there were always tasty options to eat when eating at home.

Regarding how I felt physically, I still think my body needs animal protein. Even though there were no effects on my training capacity, sleep, intestinal regularity, or overall mood, I felt a bit off kilter and unenergized, especially in the last week of this challenge.

It was the first time since I started these food experiments that people commented on how tired I looked. Which often with the Portuguese, means you look old. Of course my less than fresh look could be for many reasons, including that I have lost a significant amount of weight throughout the year and it may be becoming noticeable on my 51-year-old face.

Also, I have stopped dying my hair over the past year, so it is now full grey especially at the front. And finally, the last few weeks have not been easy for personal reasons, which means I am likely carrying a bit of pain on my face. Glad I did it? Yes! Will I continue? No! Will it change how I eat? Yes.

Similarly to all the other challenges, this month will likely have a long-term impact on what the whole family eats, even if it is simply the introduction of foods that were not a part of our household before. Here are the positives and negatives as I see them:

Positives
- Once again, explored with new foods.
- Found a fantastic authentic Chinese supermarket in downtown Lisbon, with great different veggies and spices.
- Reveled in various nut butters, such as cashew, peanut, sesame, and almond.
- Lost 1 kg in 1 month.
- Lost 1 cm waist circumference.
- Regular bowel and intestinal movements.
- Felt ok at the gym and at training (although there were no competitions during this time).
- Could drink beer and wine.
- Vegan was easier to do than I thought.
- Very affordable diet, especially when compared to paleo.

Negatives
- I really do not like having food limitations, and find that these impose non healthy choices. This is a recurring theme, and it feels fantastic to think that this month was the last time I will have to live with limitations for a while since the last challenge of the year will be about time restrictions rather than restrictions on what I can eat.
- Parties and social gatherings were extremely difficult.
- I found it too easy to get really drunk too quickly because of food limitations.

- Vegan can lead to junky eating, as there are a lot of vegan unhealthy foods including all sugars, chips, french-fries, ketchup, corn chips and corn based products, processed soy products, etcetera.
- This diet lacks essential nutrients, such as vitamin B12, fish fats and creatine, which I believe are important for my best mind/body self.

My day off

I started the day with the much dreamt about cheese and vegetable omelet, which tasted absolutely amazing! And for dinner, I made fish soft tacos with guacamole that were oh so yum. Happy to be vegan free!

In retrospect

As I finish editing the vegan month and re-live the experience, I realize that I have something emotionally against this diet. In all fairness, and with complete respect for some good friends that enjoy a healthy vegan lifestyle, I don't feel good after a few weeks without eating animal protein. Although my diet is mostly plant-based, I consider dairy, eggs and fish to be an integral part of my regular foods. Also, I seriously crave red meat after an intense training session or a long day of playing beach ultimate, and I love to follow my instincts.

There is obviously a lot to be improved in our corrupt and destructive intense farming practices, food distribution methods, labeling legislation, and impressive food waste. We throw approximately 40 % of what we produce in the garbage, and this in a planet where many suffer from hunger.

But independently of these bad production practices, we are an omnivorous species and I think we should be eating a wide variety of foods. I do try to buy organic eggs and other animal produce, as well as bring home the whole chicken from the grocery store, rather than just the chicken breasts. I hope that not supporting intense non-organic farming with these types of measures helps in re-adjusting the balance away from mass production and towards smaller more sustainable approaches to farming.

I believe in quality foods, and despair at the fact that quality is often directly proportional to price, which results in many people not having the healthy choice. It is highly frustrating to see the huge contrast in price between expensive wholesome and affordable processed foods. And this social injustice is more extreme in the western developed world. Think about it in terms of eating dinner out. What cheap healthy options are there that allow for feeding an entire family the number of calories equivalent to those that are found in a burger and fries, or pizza, for the same or less cost?

There is absolutely no doubt in my mind that our current food system is detrimental to our health as well as the health of our planet and that a shift towards a more plant based diet would be greatly beneficial.

For a comprehensive analysis comparing the estimated economic and health benefits of diet shifts towards the healthy guidelines, vegetarian or vegan, I highly recommend taking a look at Springmann et al 2016 and the references therein.

In summary, it is currently estimated that the food industry is responsible for more than a quarter of all greenhouse gas emissions, with up to 80 % of these being associated with livestock production. Compared with a reference scenario for the year 2050, a transition towards more plant-based diets could reduce global mortality by 6–10 % and food-related greenhouse gas emissions by 29–70 %. This translates into an estimated economic benefit 1–31 trillion US dollars, which is equivalent to 0.4–13 % of global gross domestic product (GDP) in 2050.

I strongly believe it is important to be cognizant of the issues associated with our food industry, especially in the developed world where processed fast food is quick to grab and always the cheapest option. As always, knowledge is key, and we can all make a difference on our health as well as the health of our planet by the choices we make.

To end on a lighter note, I the vegan experience reminds me of Kate, a PhD colleague of mine at the university in Toronto who lived as a vegetarian for 51 out of 52 weeks per year. For one week of the year, she enjoyed hunting and eating meat while camping in the great Canadian wilderness.

In the end, I am very happy at the fact that I completed this challenge. Once again, the capacity to stick to it resulted in increased self-trust and a sense of accomplishment. I also realized throughout this challenge that I had developed a solid and strong will-power.

Vegan revisited – November 2018

I have expanded my vegan culinary experience in the past two years, and have had the pleasure of enjoying some excellent vegan meals. Not only at home, but also at some great restaurants that have popped up recently. *Massive Roots* is one of my faves, a fantastic breakfast and lunch place in Estoril recently opened by my health coach, Patricia, and her partner. Food the way nature meant it to be and wonderful to the palate.

Regarding whether I consider vegan a healthy lifestyle option, the answer is not without supplementation if it is done long-term (more than 3 years). Any food regimen that requires supplementation is not complete and a complete nourishing diet from nature is ideal. That said, we store vitamin B12 in the liver for years and our need for it can be met by eating eggs, dairy, sea foods or insects very occasionally.

References

Springmann M, Godfray HCJ, Rayner M, Scarborough P. 2016. Analysis and valuation of the health and climate change cobenefits of dietary change. Proceedings of the National Academy of Sciences, Vol. 113, pp. 4146

Chapter 12 – intermittent fasting

Wow! What a strange feeling to realize that the twelfth and final challenge is here and that 30 days from now I will be finished one full year of food experiments. For this final month, I will be doing intermittent fasting and am looking forward to it. Especially because rather than having restrictions on what I can eat, this challenge will be about time, meaning that I will only be able to eat for a limited amount of time each day.

There are many reasons why I chose to do intermittent fasting as my last experiment. As you have likely heard somewhere on social media or in the press, there is a lot of interest in the health benefits of periodically going without food for some time. In fact, it has repeatedly been shown that fasting significantly increases longevity in various animal species, mainly by slowing down metabolism.

For us humans, the positive health effects of diets that impose lengthened periods of caloric restriction have turned fasting regimes into a business, as exemplified in https://www.fastcompany.com/3068951/the-business-of-fasting.

I personally have used periodical fasting for 24 hours as a reset, and fully believe in the power of these fasts on the health of my body and brain. If you think about it, various forms of fasting are a part of most of our religions and traditions throughout the ages.

Regarding fasting regimes, the one that I will be following is similar to what is practiced by Muslims during the holy month of Ramadan, when eating food, drinking liquids, smoking cigarettes, and engaging in any sexual activity is out of bounds between sunrise to sunset.

For the next month, I will follow a strict daily fasting and feasting regime where I can eat for 8 hours out of every 24 hours. My regime will be somewhat similar to the fasting practiced by Muslims during Ramadan, yet different in terms of day/night restrictions. My 16 hours without food will include the nightly sleep hours.

To start, I intend to stick to a schedule of being able to eat between 12 and 8 pm, and starve between 8 pm and 12 pm of the following day. However, I will also allow for flexibility in the schedule to be able to adjust for special occasions, such as a night in which there is a dinner party.

In order to alter the schedule, I must extend the fasting time to more than 16 hours or shorten the feasting time. This means that I can always shorten the amount of time I can eat, but shortening the fasting time will not be permitted. Unlike during Ramadan, I will be able to drink water, teas, infusions, and black coffee during the 16 hours of fasting, but cannot ingest any calories.

There are many fasting regimes with various daily or weekly fasting/feasting schedules, such as fasting every other day, one day a week, etcetera. I chose this regime completely intuitively, as it seemed not too difficult to follow while still imposing a good daily fast. But I realized after googling "eat 8 hours fast 16 hours" that this is probably the simplest and most recommended fasting method for a beginner.

The absolute pleasure of this challenge is that I will be able to eat anything I feel like. The fact that I can only eat for 8 hours will likely make my choices more important to me, so I am curious as to how I will choose what to eat and how much I eat.

Also, I wonder if I can "listen to my body" regarding my eating choices. And even if I do eat well, I worry about whether I will be able to keep myself energetic and feeling good through the fasting periods. Sixteen hours without eating is a lot of time to be on an empty stomach and capable of working, training, playing disc, having fun, and so on.

But this is the final challenge! During this month, I am very curious to see how this year has widened my choices of what I eat. I wonder what I will learn. And although I am looking forward to it, I am also slightly worried about hungry grumpy mornings.

My anxiety level starts to rise at the idea of going an entire month without my much-loved late night hot milk (or vegetable milk) with cinnamon, especially after nightly training sessions,. Add to that, I am slightly concerned about the quality of my sleep, as I tend to sleep badly on an empty stomach. Let us see how it goes.

Day 1

It is now almost eleven o'clock in the morning on the first day of fasting, and although I feel like I have lots of energy, I am starving! Last night, after a couple of hours of disc training on the beach, I enjoyed a nice cold after-practice beer, the last for the next month. Then I came home and had a late-night snack before going to bed, which means that right now, I am nowhere near 16 hours without food.

I am curious as to how difficult it is going be to have the last food before disc practice, and then eventually go to bed five or six hours later and on an empty stomach. And then after I wake up in the morning, I am not sure how am I expected to function for so many hours without eating. Longer-term, I wonder how this regime is going to impact my physical strength, which is decent at this point due to regular strength training and plenty of disc.

According to what is currently known, a healthy meal containing protein is beneficial after training, as it promotes muscle synthesis which in turn is important to repair exercise-induced muscle damage as well as for building muscle mass. I am thinking about this and considering what is the best way to adjust my training schedules this month to make sure I avoid injuries or regression in performance.

But first, I must get through today, which means at least one more hour before I can eat! Best to get busy, so I will use the time to walk to the village to take care of some banking and then go take a look at what the butcher has to offer for my first meal of the day. Steak for breakfast seems like a good way to enjoy my first red meat meal in over a month, and a perfect choice considering that I am starving and ready for some cave-woman food and feeding!

Forty-five minutes later on the clock and I am now back from the village with a bag full of chicken legs wrapped up in typical Portuguese sausage (farinheira) and bacon to put into the oven for about an hour. Funny that it was the most attractive food at the butcher, even compared to steaks or meat stuffed Portobello mushrooms. I was surprised by my choice.

I think what turned me off the mushrooms was the cheese on top. My relationship with cheese has changed, especially lower quality cheeses commonly used in restaurants and other prepared food establishments, which are only partially made with dairy and often have potato starch in them. No longer the unconditional love it used to be, or at least a more selective unconditional love.

Day 2

Exactly what I was afraid that would happen did happen, and last night I woke up in the middle of the night very unhappy and very hungry. It took me a long time to go back to sleep, and in the morning I got out of bed heavy headed and frustrated at the realization that I had to wait at least three hours before I could eat.

To add insult to injury, my stomach is not feeling great. It could be because of the different animal foods I ate yesterday or perhaps it is the eating/fasting regime itself. A green tea helped ease the pain in my upper abdomen, but this is not going to be easy and I am starting to doubt if I can do it. Odd that after successfully completing almost an entire year of challenges, I still have doubts if I can manage to complete this month.

Day 4

It is again morning and I am again crazy with hunger. Thinking beyond the hunger, I feel like my brain is highly functioning, similarly as to how it was during the ketogenic month. That makes me wonder if having undergone 30 ketogenic days in the not too distant past has helped my body and brain to be quicker to adapt to burning fat for energy.

There are many things running through my mind and my mind's mind at this point, from simple and practical things like food to more complex ones like evolution and the nervous system. I hope I don't bore you as I let my brain and fingers go loose and write. More importantly, and considering my feverish and frantic food deprived state, I hope that my writing makes sense.

One thing is for sure, and that is that right now I am not happy. Not only am I grumpy hungry, I also have a lingering and irritating dull pain in my upper abdominal area, which seems to persist after settling in on day one of this starvation regime. I talked about this pain to a friend who regularly lives with this fasting regime and he doesn't recognize this symptom in himself. Yet, although he has never felt fast induced pain, for me it is real.

I can localize the pain with my fingers to my stomach and upper intestine, and attribute it to their having to adjust to being empty for such long periods of time. Also, for the first time in all these months of doing various dietary regimes, my intestines are seriously suffering, my bowel movements have not been pleasant, and I have had a fair bit of gas. A self-imposed scatological mess, is what it is!

In reality, I don't know how to manage the fact that there are still many hours to go before I can eat. Although I have periodically done 24 hour fasting bouts before and know what it feels like to be seriously hungry and have an empty stomach, there is a big difference between those isolated experiences and the feeling you get after consecutive days of 16 hours with no food. Now, when I think about it, I recall having a seriously upset stomach for a few days following my last 24-hour starvation bout.

To help the time go by, I should focus on what I can learn from this experience. From a psychological and physiological perspective, I am interested in the frantic over-aware state that I am in, which is likely induced by my unhappy empty stomach and intestinal tract as well as a constant state of hunger. Let me take you on a trip into our gut and let us talk about the scoop on poop.

If we think about it, our digestive system is like a tube that travels from our heads to our butts. It is a complex tube with many different compartments and physiological environments, including the mouth, the esophagus, the stomach, the small intestine, the large intestine, the colon, bowel, rectum... etcetera. In our well-fed western society, this tube is hardly ever completely empty of food or its remnants.

In fact, a significant portion of the remnants of food that we can't digest ourselves serve to feed the trillions of micro-organisms that live in our gut. Regarding my unpleasant bowel movements, I am now convinced that fasting is inducing drastic changes in the highly complex population of bacteria, viruses, archaea and fungi that live in my gut. It makes sense, and partially explains my current discomfort I feel as my gut community adjusts to the shock treatment imposed by this regime.

To put it simply, my gut's microbiota and the pool of DNA and genes that these micro-organisms synthetize need time to adapt to the new unfed and mostly empty environment at the end of my tube. The good news is that I believe adaptation is under way, since I finally had a semi-normal dump today after a few days of serious gases, diarrhea, and mucus yuck-ness. Fingers crossed that it is the end of an unhappy intestinal time.

On top of an unsettled belly and frantic brain, intermittent fasting is having other effects on me. For one thing, I think it is influencing my autonomic nervous system, which is the part of the nervous system that we can't control. Somehow, I feel that there must be a physical reason to the heightened awareness and slightly agitated over-awake state of mind that I am in.

Bear with me a moment as I go through my off-the-cuff divagations on this and try to make sense of my current over-very hungry mental/physical state. Our autonomic nervous system has a "flight and fight" mode (sympathetic) and the "rest and digest" mode (parasympathetic). My question is, in what mode of our nervous system fits the state in which getting food is the one sole priority?

In my view, this is almost an intermediate state, where

there is a "fight and forage" energetic need as well as a "calm down and preserve" whatever energy stores you currently have. This mode, essential for survival, I will call the "I must get food" mode, and am sure that it has been a part of our existence and the existence of our predecessors since way before we evolved into a species.

To end this entry, that is precisely the mode I am in right now. In truth, I am feeling slightly overwhelmed as the "I must get food" mode completely takes over my body/brain, and so will try to focus on reading up on the effects of fasting on the autonomic nervous system until it is time to eat.

Day 5

On the fifth day of fasting and thankfully today I woke up feeling a little more normal. Perhaps there is hope that I am getting used to the empty feeling in my abdomen.

On a practical level and from an anthropological point of view, it is interesting to see how tough intermittent fasting is to stick to, even after eleven challenges. Unlike during previous limits that were based exclusively on what I could eat and not how much to eat, I am often very hungry and cannot eat.

On the other hand, I've had to force myself to eat when I was not hungry, as was the case last night. Even though I did not feel like eating just before 8 pm, knowing that 16 hours of fasting was coming made eating a must. In the end, it's a good thing that I did force myself to eat something, since right now, using a phrase commonly uttered in the laboratory by an Australian post-doc from my PhD days, I could eat the crotch out of a rag doll.

On a positive note, it seems like my intestines and their normal rhythms are getting back on track, and I no longer feel the unhappy and protesting intestinal tract and painful stomach of the past days. Probably because I do feel better, even though I am bonkers-hungry, I am much more positive today and curiously looking forward to seeing how this month goes.

One thing that I now realize is that I have to schedule my days differently, and avoid making important appointments in the mornings before I am allowed to eat. For example, tonight I have disc practice from 9 to 11 pm. Since my last meal will be before 8 pm, I will be on an empty stomach when I go to sleep tonight. And then, I will have to function tomorrow morning for hours without food.

A Muslim friend who does Ramadan every year just reached out, and mentioned that he has played entire disc tournaments of up to three matches in a day without a morsel of food or a drop of water. It is amazing the immensity of the power of our brains, where the perception of effort can be just as prejudicial as the actual physical demand.

Speaking of brains, I have accumulated a decently thick stack of science papers on the biological effects of fasting to go through. I am looking forward to digging in, and considering that I have the excuse that I worked hard today, and there could be worse and less productive things I could be doing.

When I start to think about all this reading and writing, and the possibility of publishing, I worry whether the content of this book will be interesting for you the reader. Those thoughts are not worth dwelling into, since I can't change them now. The one thing that I do like is that I will be self-publishing, which means that I can adjust or change things later, depending on your feedback, if there is feedback.

Ok, off to study what is happening in my body.

Day 6

Intermittent fasting imposes some serious changes in the way that I eat as well as in what I eat. So far, I have mostly been eating high protein and fat meals with some fresh greens and fruits. Almost like paleo but also including high quality full fat yogurts and full fat cheese. I have had one stinky cheese meal, but otherwise no major cravings for cheese. I have also been eating whole grains, mostly oats in yogurt. About the scheduling of my meals, I am still working on it.

I have noticed that I eat way too much in my first meal at around mid-day and then as a result am not hungry again until late afternoon. This means that at around 4 or 5 pm, when I am hungry again, I eat a second meal and do not feel like eating again when it is time to have my last meal before the 16-hour fasting bout.

Since fasting is not yet completely natural to me, I have to force myself to consciously be aware and adjust my eating. For one thing, I find it difficult to chew slowly and to leisurely enjoy my first meal of the day when I am ravenous after so many hours of fasting.

The other lesson to be learnt is the scheduling of meals themselves. For example, last night after lazy Sunday pickup I realized walking home from the beach that I had 15 minutes before the fasting bout. I ended up running into a small Chinese supermarket and buying an avocado and sesame snaps and quickly chowing down an impromptu plain guacamole made of hand squished avocado scooped up by sesame snaps. Not a bad combination, by the way.

Day 7

I just finished my first meal of the day and it is now almost 2 pm. Breakfast for lunch or lunch for breakfast consisted of eggs, veggies and some whole grain bread. Perhaps because of a friend being over to share breakfast/lunch, or perhaps because of the realization yesterday that I wanted to postpone my 8 hours eating time by one hour (from 12-8 pm to 1-9 pm) to adjust feasting time to end just after sunset, I actually enjoyed preparing the meal before sitting down with everyone to eat it.

And today it happened easily and organically... I only started eating after 17 hours of fasting and one hour after the time I was allowed to start. Also, I am proud to say that I managed to chew and eat slowly regardless of my hunger. In fact, I somehow managed to have been the last one of the three people at the meal table to have food on my plate.

Funny how little things can feel like such large achievements. Since cheating is out of the question this late in the game, it is important for me to be able to enjoy food for the rest of this challenge, and I am happy to be getting into the swing of things.

Today, for the first time since I started this challenge, I will focus on making sure that I have three decent meals during my 8 food-ok hours. Big meal first, small something when I get hungry later on in the afternoon, and then a larger meal at night. That should work better than what I have been doing. Although I have done very little physical activity, in general I feel good. Brain is on. Like in Keto.

Day 8

Starting to feel closer to normal. The toughest part of this challenge are the mornings, where I have to wait 4 or 5 hours after I wake up before I can eat. On a positive note, the fact that food is a no-no frees up a load of time.

Also, although I did not mention it before, my menstrual cycle is completely screwed up, having started about 10 days ago, then intermittently coming and going until now. I wonder if this is partially because of the vegan month, where I used a load of soy products, including tofu, fresh soy sprouts and tempeh, for cooking. What is more likely is that these irregularities are normal pre-menopausal symptoms, taking into account my current 51 going on 52 years. Anyway, I thought I would mention it.

Although I feel much better today, this week has not been easy. Even right now, I have a hollow feeling in my gut and my stomach feels unusually heavy while empty at the same time. At around 14 hours of no food, my needy stomach has gotten to the point of pain, but I can function and not think about it if I get busy.

Before going off to live my day, there is one more thing that has been frequently on my mind in the last days. This challenge has made me realize that I spend way too much time focused on food or food related issues. The "hungry human" is probably how we have frequently existed and persisted throughout evolution, where hunger was our normal state.

Even nowadays, the majority of people in the developing world go through their daily lives hungry. Perhaps because of the partially fast induced ketogenic state of my brain as well as the "heightened awareness" that comes from not having anything in my stomach, I am thinking a lot about this.

Let me boldly put it out there... here goes... from a social and economic perspective, maybe the western world would have something to gain if we all went through this experience, maybe we should all be going hungry more often.

Day 9

Today, I am amazed at how normal it feels to now go 16 or 17 hours without eating. After one week and a half of fasting, I am finally feeling good. I get the sensation of having gotten used to this regime - by mainly maintaining a low rhythm of activity in the mornings when I am most hungry and starting to carry out more physical activities after my first meal around 1 pm.

Tomorrow morning I plan to go to the gym with my

daughter Sara to do a Zumba class at 11, and am curious as to how energetic or lethargic I will feel dancing while starving. Yesterday, I noticed that I have to be careful about how much I eat, as I think that I started eating a bit too much during the 8 feasting hours.

I have to stay away from highly caloric not great-for-me stuff like typical Portuguese cream pastries (pastel de nata), chips, or ice-cream. After a few bad "giving in to cravings" days, yesterday and today things are back to normal and I am eating healthy foods from all food groups and natural sources.

I am particularly loving eggs with lots of veggies. In a way, this challenge reminds me of the ketogenic and paleo challenges, as I often choose to eat high fat and protein meals that are low in carbs, especially towards the end of the day.

Day 10

Over the last week, I have been enjoying digesting a small part of the huge amount of scientific literature available on the topic of intermittent fasting. I have yet to find a negative health effect of intermittent fasting. On the other hand, there are so many benefits that it's hard to know where to start.

From stimulating stem cell regeneration to inducing increased insulin sensitivity (which is a serious problem in our society and results in type 2 diabetes), the health promoting effects of fasting are widespread and overwhelming. I also found that there are significant similarities and overlaps between the positive outcomes of intermittent fasting, high intensity exercise and ketogenic and/or paleo low carb diets.

Although I am not a huge fan of "conspiracy theories", such as those imposed on the food industry convincing us to eat much more and many more times a day than we need, I do like the energetic and mentally aware state that comes from what I call a "keto brain", loosely meaning a brain that is adapted to being powered by fats instead of carbs.

For a great video discussing the effects of fasting on brain function, I strongly suggest taking the time to see a TEDx entitled "Why fasting bolsters brain power", by Mark Mattson from Johns Hopkins University (link: www.youtube.com/watch?v=4UkZAwKoCP8).

Day 12

After almost two weeks, I am now moving well through this challenge and surprisingly enjoying it. I feel physically good and strong, sleep surprisingly well, have lots of energy, and as I already mentioned repeatedly, I feel clear-headed and my brain is sharp.

Regarding food, I am now eating well in the 8 hours which I am allowed to eat, and likely come close to consuming the approximately 2000 calories that I normally eat on a day. This is supported by my weight, which so far remains exactly the same as it was at the beginning of this challenge.

My son, Tomas, who would like to lose some kilograms, has decided to join me on this regime for two weeks, and is going on to his second day today. He seems to be sliding easily into it, partially because he is on Easter holidays and therefore has no schedule and sleeps in quite late.

Tomorrow, I do have a challenge within this challenge, as I have to do an oral presentation at the library in Cascais a couple of hours before I can start to eat. I am curious as to how that will go, and whether I will be able to maintain focus, energy and positivity throughout my talk and during the discussion period afterwards.

Day 13

Being "on" at the presentation that I gave in the Cascais library at 10:30 am this morning was not an easy feat. Even before leaving home, I had to dig deep within to be in a good place and have the energy that my audience deserved from me. But in truth, after eating my last meal at 8 pm yesterday and training afterwards, I was grumpy hungry and drained.

I don't think that the people that were there to listen to me felt it, I found it very tiring and a bit demanding to talk about healthy fats to a full room while being on an empty stomach for more than 14 hours.

Today was one of those days that I seriously questioned myself for doing these experiments. I wanted to eat desperately. Period. Once again, I did get through it and am alive and well. One more chalked down to experience. Even though I have now eaten and am not hungry grumpy, I am still not in the best of moods.

Day 18

It is now 9:23 in the morning and I am so hungry that I

keep thinking about that Australian post-doc again, and his rag dolls. It has been over 16 hours since I have eaten, and hopefully I can last without suffering too much.

At least another three hours until I dig my chops into that yummy yogurt with banana, nuts and peanut butter which has been nicely maturing overnight in the fridge. Sixteen hours gone and three more to go means a total of 19 hours of fasting! Why so long? you may ask. And the answer is that I have to adjust back to a normal feeding time of 1 to 9 pm after a beach ultimate National league day yesterday.

Our team played four games and since I wanted to make sure I could run around starting at 9:30 in the morning, I stopped eating at 5 pm two afternoons ago (a Saturday) so that I could start eating at 9 am yesterday, before the first game. Taking into account that I can only eat for 8 hours, my last meal was at 5 pm yesterday, just after the last game. So, even though 16 hours of fasting have passed and technically I am allowed to eat, I will try to go as long as I can without food to go back to a decent eating schedule and eat dinner with my family tonight.

Intermittent fasting and my decision to alter the hours for the frisbee day ended up posing a couple of interesting challenges. For one, after my last meal at 5 pm on Saturday afternoon two days ago, Patrick, the kids and I went to see the football game at a bar close by. It was great to hang out with my grownup kids while all three drank a cold draft beer and enjoyed typical Portuguese snacks called "tremoços" (salted lupines).

However, my hot herbal tea just did not cut it as far as the enjoyment factor goes.

The next day was game day, and excluding some energy breaks especially in the third game that I think were felt by everyone else on the team as well, I felt ok. My tiredness at the end of the day may have nothing to do with the current challenge, and was surely at least partially explained by the hot sunny day as well as the fact that we only had four women, which means I played every other point throughout the day.

There is a lot of interest in fasting and how it influences physical and athletic capacity, and I have included key references at the end of this chapter. According to a comprehensive review by Shephard (2012), there are very small, if any, effects of Ramadan on explosive capacity (anaerobic power), measured as sprint speed.

There are, however, small but significant fasting induced effects on fatigue, shown as a slight yet significant decrease in performance in comparison to fed controls over repetitive runs. These results are further discussed by the authors, who mention the importance of keeping in mind that the tendency towards greater fatigue with event repetition may be attributable to sleep deprivation or a phase shift in the intake of food in Ramadan fasting athletes, rather than to a cumulative nutritional impairment.

Regarding muscle contractile force, the intermittent fasting regime imposed by Ramadan appears to have small effects, especially if hydration, training times and resting times are controlled. Therefore, and taken together, the studies indicate that if sleep patterns are not disrupted and training is maintained, there is little change of anaerobic power or capacity over the month of Ramadan.

That brings me to another interesting parameter that is affected by fasting, brain function and perception. I must admit that this regime has chiseled away at my patience. This was obvious to me during the first beach ultimate game yesterday, which was against a tough opponent and my team played horribly. Even though I am usually positive and supporting, I felt like smacking a few of my teammates and had to take deep breaths to control my temper.

There is no doubt that this type of negativity can have an influence on athletic performance. In fact, it appears that fasting has effects on perceived exertion, mood profile including fatigue, as well as the amount of perceived energy demands by the athletes. Ramadan-style fasting also seems to affect psychomotor performance and vigilance, evident as decreased alertness and concentration.

The science indicates that these negative effects are directly associated to the number of hours of fasting, aggravating as the number of fasting hours increase. Regarding my state during games, I felt highly aware of what was going on at all times. But, I have noticed that I have to put more mental effort into focusing while working out in the last two weeks, a feeling that is somewhat reminiscent from that which I felt while doing the ketogenic challenge.

Conversely to what has been shown for anaerobic

power and performance, where athletes show little Ramadan-related deterioration, there is significant deterioration of performance in longer bouts of endurance (aerobic) exercises. It remains unclear whether this is due to poorer motivation, depletion of glycogen reserves, or progressive dehydration.

Perhaps this data is related to the increasing fatigue that I feel as the day passes, resulting in lethargic lazy evenings. Reminiscent to how I felt on the ketogenic diet, I am tired after sunset and have to force myself to be active. To sum up how I felt yesterday, during a sports day, I must admit that I didn't feel my best on day 17 of intermittent fasting, although I also definitely did not feel my worst.

As I mentioned earlier in this entry, due to my decision to eat before the games started in the morning, my last meal yesterday was at 5 pm just after the games, and consisted of a large hamburger and a cold beer. Sadly not enough, and I was already feeling an uncomfortably empty stomach and a huge desire to eat just a few hours later. A horrible feeling that was exacerbated by watching my kids and husband eating dinner.

Well if you can imagine, hungry then and ravenous now... although I still have a couple of hours to go. Got to get busy cleaning drawers or doing something else mundane but useful. I can't concentrate and am getting grumpy, so perhaps I will go for a walk and pick up some necessities.

Now a few hours have gone by and I am back, feeling proud of myself, and just about to ingest my first calories in over 19 hours. But first a few words. I was having a very hard time focusing because of hunger and decided to walk up to the village and pick up some veggies for a soup. When 12 o'clock hit, which is the time I could start eating, I was in the grocery store. Boy I was tempted to buy a pastry or something to quickly shove in my mouth. But no, I hung in there…

When I got home, I started cooking a veggie soup with fresh fava beans and am now sitting down writing these few words before getting my overnight yogurt out of the fridge, which I am now about to eat. Going to focus on enjoying it, chewing slowly and not devouring my first meal in close to 20 hours.

Day 20

Dinner last night with the book-club ladies was interesting and indicative of how socially difficult this regime can be. Since our dinners typically start around 9 pm, I opted to eat before going and sat and drank tea as everyone else ate.

None of the ladies even flinched, as they are now used to my monthly gustatory insanities. On a good note, it turned out to be easier than I thought, likely due to the fact that there are only 10 days to go until I am done.

Day 22

Last night, while lying in bed, I was thinking about the reasons why I don't like fasting and made a conscious decision to write things down this morning while they were fresh in my mind.

I am aware that fasting is good it for me in the sense

that it makes the good bacteria in my gut flourish while getting rid of the unhealthy ones, gets rid of cells and cell parts in my system that have accumulated mutations, reduces inflammation, and protects against neurodegeneration. But the truth is that I feel various negative effects, which seem to get worse as time goes by.

For one thing, I am eating much more junky food than I normally do in the 8 hours that I can eat. Partially due to hunger desperation and partially because of psychological factors, I tend to look towards floury high calorie stuff much more often and then think "it's ok, you won't be eating for 16 hours, go for it!". It will be interesting to see how much I weigh at the end of this challenge, but right now I would say that I have not lost any weight at all.

Another negative aspect of fasting is the fact that my mornings are highly unproductive. I generally wake up between 7 and 8 am and can only eat my first meal between 12 and 1 pm. Truthfully, I find that after being awake for two or three hours in the morning, I cannot concentrate on my work due to hunger issues.

To add to the negative aspects, I don't feel the energy for using this "unproductive" time to exercise because I am too hungry. In the end, I find myself doing mundane things like cleaning up around the house until I can eat. Also negative is the fact that once I do eat, I feel a bit too full to be at my best. But at least I can focus. Yet one more significant issue that I don't like about intermittent fasting is that I am not my sunny self. At least in the mornings and late at nights, I find that I am grumpy. Hungry grumpy, or grumpy hungry. My husband has mentioned it too, and I also notice it in my son who is also fasting with me. He is quicker to explode than when in his usual mode, even considering that he is 16 and volatile.

Day 26

Today marks the one year anniversary since I started this craziness, and to be honest, I am starting to get tired of challenges and cannot wait to be able to eat normally again.

My son has decided that two weeks was enough for him, mostly because he had trouble focusing in his morning classes on an empty stomach. He did, however, lose 700 g in two weeks. Regarding my weight, I have no idea what it is but would bet that I haven't lost one gram so far. As far as this challenge goes, I am now decidedly not enjoying intermittent fasting.

One of the things I most detest about this regime is the constant stress around time. The having to be aware of what time it is right now, when is the time that I can start eating and how long can I eat for, is driving me mad. I have always hated being attached to the clock, avoided living by strict schedules ... thus my choice to be a researcher and now to work as a health-coach.

Just the imposing presence of a time limit on my eating makes me unproductive and unhappy. But again, there is a huge amount of discipline involved and that is good. My anarchic self needs it.

Concerning what I am eating when I do eat, the quality of foods in what I choose to eat has improved significantly this week. I am making a conscious effort to think about the decisions I make and not hang onto the "well, I'm not going to eat for hours and hours, so anything goes" kind of mentality.

Last week, I found that I was getting uncomfortable stomach gases and feeling bloated. After a few days with no dairy and very little wheat, all went back to normal. It is interesting that excluding the first adaptation week, there seem to be no effects of this regime on the frequency of my going to the bathroom.

Day 29

Oh my, I am almost done! And not only this challenge, but a full year of challenges. And oh boy, it will end with a bang! A verified smorgasbord! Why, you may ask? Well, tonight we have my friend's kid from Toronto and his friend staying at our place and we are going out for a celebratory seafood dinner accompanied by cold beers in a traditional Portuguese "tasca" style restaurant.

This means that I won't start eating until around 3 pm today so that I can enjoy a typically late Portuguese dinner. And then tomorrow we are going to my cousin's wedding - another late-night feast that starts at the church around 4 pm.

Similarly to today, I will only start eating late into the afternoon tomorrow, so that I don't have to think about it anymore. Once midnight hits, I am done! All done!

Tomorrow will be crazy busy with the guests staying

over as well as the wedding, and Sunday will not be a good day to measure anything after pigging out, so I did my metrics today. This morning I weighed in at 55.6 Kg and my waist circumference was 76 cm.

Considering the logistics of this coming weekend (today is Friday), this is probably the last time that I will be doing a daily log. The feeling is strange, I almost feel queasy at the thought that it is over, nerves mixed with elation and a sense of pride. I can't believe I did it!

More than one year has gone by and I am almost free of food limitations. What will happen next? How will this experience affect my eating choices in the future? What about my weight? And how will I use different types diets at specific times of life and for achieving specific objectives like muscle building, weight loss or a high functioning mind?

Conclusion

After an entire year of doing food challenges, I had no doubt that I could get through this challenge without cheating, no matter how tough it was or how desperate I got.

The fact that the limitations this month were about when I ate rather than what I ate, fasting turned out to be the perfect ending to a fantastic 12-month journey of food experiments. After 30 days, I can clearly state that I am not an advocate of this regime as a lifestyle choice. I do, however, think it is a great way to reset your body, to train self-discipline, or to shake up your relationship with food.

Regarding my weight, no significant differences

occurred this month (I lost 100 g) and to be honest, I think it is probably the month that I ate the least healthy of out of the entire last year. Partially, this can be explained by my own internal voice, which excused me to eat whatever I wanted during "feast" hours with the excuse that a long time of hunger was coming up. On top of that, the excessive hunger I felt after 16 fast hours often resulted in over indulging.

Many times, during my first meals of the day, I would be eating and desperately thinking of what I was going to eat after I finished what I had on my plate. Crazy with hunger, literally. And, I ate way too much for my last meal before the time to fast, just knowing I wouldn't be eating for a long time. For me, this does not seem to be a healthy routine.

Another issue with this fasting regime is that it is socially very difficult. There were many complaints from my husband regarding the lack of flexibility in eating hours and grumpiness. There were also various dinners and social gatherings that I went to and did not eat or drink. The difficulty of sticking to a fasting regime is recognized in the scientific literature. The data indicates that the number of drop-outs is greater in fasting than for other caloric restriction diet regimes.

The effects of fasting on weight loss, fat content and cardio-protective parameters have been the subject of many scientific studies, as reviewed in Harvie and Howell, 2016. Analysis of the long-term effects of fasting recently published in one of the most prestigious medical journals (JAMA) showed that alternate-day fasting did not produce superior adherence, weight loss, weight maintenance, or cardio-protection in comparison to regimes of daily calorie restriction.

These conclusions were further supported by data of shorter term studies accumulated over the last years, which concluded that intermittent fasting and general calorie restriction diets result in comparable reductions in body weight as well as equivalent reductions in body fat. One exception was observed when the intermittent fasting regime was also a very low carb (50 g a day) and high fat diet, in which case there was a greater decrease in body fat when fasting.

Fasting, however, has many beneficial effects on inflammation, brain function, immune system, etcetera. It will be interesting to keep up to the scientific literature as knowledge increases regarding the long-term effects of fasting.

Personally, I have no doubt that periodic bouts of intermittent fasting can be very positive, having effects in cleansing, resetting, and as a shock to the system. In fact, emerging findings strongly suggest that periodic fasting, together with exercise and an intellectually challenging lifestyle, can protect neurons against the dysfunction and degeneration that they would otherwise suffer in acute brain injuries such as stroke and head trauma, as well as against neurodegenerative disorders including Alzheimer's, Parkinson's and Huntington's disease.

However, just like all other adaptations that our bodies manage as we challenge them, after some time under the fasting stress I think our bodies get used to it and the beneficial effects are waned. In conclusion, in my opinion, we should try to keep that in mind when doing any diet of food regime. Also, it is important to remember that when it comes to food, variety and wholesomeness is key.

In conclusion, I know that I will occasionally fast, as I always have throughout my life. In fact, on the first day after this challenge and after eating way too much at the wedding, I went to the gym and did an extensive work out on an empty stomach. It felt great!

Positives
- I could eat whatever I felt like eating.
- 16 fasting hours meant that there was a lot of time to do non-food related things.
- Realized that I eat too much and too often.
- Regular bowel and intestinal movements after the first week.
- Mostly felt ok at the gym and at training, although I avoided exercise in the morning before breaking the fast.
- Huge lesson in self-discipline.
- Felt very clear headed and with a high functioning brain, especially in the first few weeks.
- Slept great, even though I was very afraid of this because I don't like going to bed hungry.

Negatives
- This was by far the most difficult challenge socially, as there are no options during fasting hours.
- Felt that I was grumpy due to hunger a lot of the time, especially in the mornings.

- Difficulty concentrating in the last few hours before eating time. Cleaned a lot of drawers and other mundane chores around the house this month.
- Ate too much crappy high calorie foods during feasting hours with the excuse that I would make up for it during fasting hours.
- Found it difficult to manage how to eat and when to eat on physical training and sports days.

My first of many days off

I have to share with you my two amazing last experiences with food as an intermittent fasting person, which were incredible feasts!

The first night, Friday night, which was the second last night in the challenge, we went for dinner at a local and well renown Portuguese sea-food place called Eduardinhos. What a wonderful way to spend the last night with Max, my close friend's kid that has been visiting for the last few weeks

We enjoyed a fantastic dinner of crab, clams, octopus salad, and sea barnacles served up with rustic Portuguese sour dough bread and accompanied by ice-cold beers. Easy and stimulating conversation with Patrick and four great teenagers while feasting on a lot of food. More than enough to make it easy to only start eating quite late on the next day, the last day of the challenge.

And then the last day, Saturday, where I only started eating after 4 pm so as not to have to think about it anymore. What a way to start... at my cousins wedding! The wedding ceremony was held in a wonderful hill-top country home with fantastic views of rolling hills and small villages, just one hour north of Lisbon.

It was by far the best served wedding I have been to in ages. The quality of the foods was amazing since it was made in-house rather than catered in. Let me just tell you, it's a good thing I weighed myself before... did I eat, and eat, and eat! Food from heaven, really.

The appetizers were served outdoors and included sushi, amazing meats, all kinds of finger foods, Portuguese smoked pork leg (presunto), and all beautiful and all wonderful and all allowed! And all served up with cocktails or your drink of choice.

Dinner was a very nice fish soup, followed by seafood crepes, and then a pork with baked apple dish. The served dinner was finalized by a desert that I did not eat. But, while dancing and talking, I thoroughly enjoyed the three large tables loaded with delicacies and kept well stacked deep into the night.

The first, and a favorite, was the cheese table. Stinky awesome cheeses that I love and that go down oh-so-well with wine. The second was a table full of high-end treats like crab, hams and smoked meats. And the third table served up all kinds of beautifully prepared deserts and fresh fruits, including one of my favorite typical Portuguese treats called "fios de ovos", which are basically egg strings made with egg yolk and sugar.

I enjoyed a couple of plates loaded with these sweet yellow strings and with fresh strawberries, pineapple, and kiwi. Heavenly and like the Dutch say, like an angel peeing on your tongue! There was so much food, that I was happy to hear that all the left-overs will be given to an association close by and then distributed to families with financial difficulties.

In retrospect

It was interesting to re-read and edit this challenge. The almost manic feeling of the first few weeks was especially obvious in the frantic writing, which I edited as little as possible.

Perhaps because it was the last of the twelve challenges, and I was therefore likely getting tired of food challenges, this challenge left a strong impression on me.

Socially, it was very difficult, as the only one of all twelve that I could not eat anything at dinners and parties. Also, I have no doubt that it was the challenge that had the biggest impact on my family, not only because of strict dinner schedules but also because it was the one that most affected my mood.

I grumpier than usual. Both kids complained that I often lost focus in a conversation and stopped sentences halfway. As far as the long-term effects of this regime on my eating, I still do not wake up and eat immediately the way that I used to, and now tend to only get hungry two or three hours after opening my eyes in the morning.

Although I will not consider this mode of eating as a long-term regime, I will use intermittent fasting periodically throughout my life to reset the body/mind. In the end, I am very glad that I chose to end the journey with this experiment, as it was a true test to my will-power and discipline.

Intermittent fasting revisited – November 2018

The biological effects of fasting or intermittent fasting are multifaceted, and we know a lot of the science, as seen in a comprehensive review published in the latest Science issue, A Time to Fast. The authors conclude with stating that the powers of fasting are worth exploring further in human health and ageing, and may provide better alternatives than drugs at times.

References

Di Francesco A, Di Germanio C, Bernier M, de Cabo R. 2018. A time to fast. Science Vol. 362, pp. 770-775

Michelle HM, Howell A. 2017. Potential Benefits and Harms of Intermittent Energy Restriction and Intermittent Fasting Amongst Obese, Overweight and Normal Weight Subjects—A Narrative Review of Human and Animal Evidence. Behavioral Sciences, Vol. 7, pp. 4

Nair PMK, Khawale PG. 2016. Role of therapeutic fasting in women's health: An overview. Journal of Mid-Life Health. Vol. 7, pp. 61

Raefsky SM, Mattson MP. 2017. Adaptive responses of neuronal mitochondria to bioenergetic challenges: Roles in neuroplasticity and disease resistance. Free Radical Biology and Medicine, Vol. 102, pp. 203

Shephard RJ. 2012. The impact of Ramadan observance upon athletic performance. Nutrients, Vol. 4, pp. 491

Trepanowski JF, Kroeger CM, Barnosky A, Klempel MC, Bhutani S, et al. 2017. Effect of Alternate-Day Fasting on Weight Loss, Weight Maintenance, and Cardioprotection Among Metabolically Healthy Obese Adults - A Randomized Clinical Trial. JAMA Internal Medicine, Published online, doi:10.1001/jamainternmed.2017.0936

Conclusions

If you have gotten this far, stop and take a slow deep breath. I just did. As we get closer to the end, I am ever more aware that writing and editing are also part of this process. And although finalizing the book is making me marginally insane and obsessive, I enjoyed re-living each challenge and seeing the whole journey evolve as the days, weeks, and months went by. For the sake of clarity, this whole portion of the book was written over a one-and-a-half-month period after the last challenge was finished, and updated science information that has been published over the last year has been added in italics.

Before I continue my prolific writing mode, I wish I could see what is going on in your mind's eye or your eye's mind. I would also love to hear about how what you have read so far has influenced your own approach to food. Has the thought of trying a food regime crossed you mind? What about trying something new when you are out food shopping or going to a specialty restaurant?

If not at all, that's ok, hopefully eventually. Regardless of your own food journeys, it is great that you are still reading. In this section, I intend to sum up the entire experience from various perspectives. Enjoy.

What Patrick and the kids thought

I am honestly not sure if I would have completed this experimental year without Patrick and the kid's encouragement and support. Living with someone with food challenges is not always easy and my husband and kids had to put up with me and my food choices for the entire year.

All three were amazing at cheering me on, giving support, and bearing with my endless talk of food and science. From my perspective, their genuine interest in the experiments and how I was doing as the best part... they were on my team throughout!

I tried not to impose my limits on them as much as possible, but considering that we have at least one daily meal together as a family, typically dinner, and that I cook a lot, our food shopping, cooking, and eating was often at the mercy of my challenges. Their feedback was constant, sometimes good and sometimes not so good.

Regarding the kids, as their mom, I would say that the most difficult thing for them was not having choices they were accustomed to because the choices themselves were always changing. Sometimes that just pissed them off. And, depending on my state, didn't make me happy either.

These less-than-ideal times were definitely worth the price of opening their horizons and expanding their comfort zone with foods. Nowadays, they often talk about funny situations throughout the challenges and appreciate the introduction of new, and much loved, ingredients of meals.

It was also great fun having them occasionally join me in the challenges, as was the case for Sara in the ovo-lacto vegetarian and the vegan months and Tomas in the intermittent fasting month. In the end, it gives me great pleasure that both the kids learnt a lot about good food, real food, and to distinguish whole foods from foods that don't exist naturally in our biological world.

Patrick was a different story, he was my buddy throughout. He was also often my filter, intellectually and emotionally. And, importantly, he encouraged me in those not so few moments that I did not think it was worthwhile to continue.

We also talked a lot of shop, and had seriously good science conversations. It's difficult to separate out all the parts, it was a whole year and we both work at home, so we share a lot.

On a practical level, Patrick was also amazing. He loves to cook and makes amazing dinners. Breakfasts and lunches are not his thing, as he is Dutch and is happy to eat yogurt and bread during the day. But he does enjoy sitting down at the table for my daytime meals, and we often have at least one of the kids at home for lunch.

Besides our shared family meals, everyone in the house loves leftovers, straight-up or re-invented. Also, we often go grocery shopping as a family. Taken together, this family lives our food together. I therefore thought it important to get their feedback on the whole experience and asked each of them three questions. Their answers follow.

Question 1 - Overall, what did you think about this year?

Patrick:

> I liked it. I thought it was interesting. I enjoyed that at times it forced me to rethink about food based on the culinary challenge of the month. That, in turn, led me to make meals I would've never have even considered. Long live Google :-)
> I also enjoyed watching Sofia go through it from a scientific point of view and grow in her knowledge. I enjoyed challenging Sof at times and learning from the responses.
> Overall, it was a very positive experience, with perhaps the exception of the last month because the fasting impeded my happy time. More about this in the answer to the next question.

Sara:

> I thought it was challenging not to be able to eat what I felt like at times because it was not in the house. For example, normal bread when mom was going through the gluten free months. But, I did find it a great learning year, and love some of the new recipes and foods we eat now, like zoodles!

Tomas:

> I found it to be interesting. It was cool trying out new foods and learning about the restrictions of specific diets.

Question 2 - Which challenge did you like the most and which one did you like the least? Why?

Patrick:

I liked all the challenges in which it wasn't easy for me to come up with a dinner meal from my usual repertoire. For these, I enjoyed going to Google and looking at what type of things I could make that I would've never thought of and that would fit Sofia's current challenge. I loved cooking those meals.

When it comes to the challenge that I liked the least, there is a clear loser for me. Fasting was by far my least favorite. Mostly because of the way I work. I get up early, work hard, and like very much what I do. But it is mentally intense, and when I'm ready to call it a day, usually around 7 pm, my happy/downtime is often to go to the kitchen and cook dinner.

I love thinking what to make and making it without deadlines, just focusing on the process. The fasting challenge completely screwed that up for me. Suddenly it was 7 pm and I knew I had to make dinner by a 7:45 because at 8 o'clock Sofia could not eat any more. That made my downtime stressful and made it my least favorite challenge, by far.

Sara:

The challenge I liked the best was paleo because I liked the foods around the house like nuts, avocados, and sweet potato cookies. The one that I liked least was ovo-lacto-vegetarian.

Since I was on summer holidays during that

experiment, I really noticed that my mom was grumpy and missing eating fish and meat. After that, things got better, maybe she got used to limits after this challenge, or maybe I just wasn't around as much because of classes.

Tomas:

The challenge I liked the most was the fasting because we went back to having no limits on the types of foods in the house and on what to make for dinner. Also, it's my favorite because I tried it myself and liked it.

In my opinion, it had good results in my weight loss and was not too difficult to do, except for focusing in my morning classes. The challenge I liked the least was ketogenic because it looked disgusting.

Question 3 - What was the biggest "take home" lesson that you got from living with a nutritionally challenged person for a year?

Patrick:

I now look at food differently. I already used to cook very internationally but this year resulted in me becoming even more open-minded. It is interesting that the challenges, which generally meant a reduction of choices, ended up increasing my culinary vocabulary and adding choices (Zoodles anyone?! :-)).

I also noticed a difference in my eating behavior because of the things that Sofia did. I have definitely incorporated more vegetables and water, while reducing bread, sugar and juices. Not necessarily because I wanted to lose weight, although that did happen, but simply knowing some of the science and theories behind foods made me want do it, and I feel good about it.

Sara:

I found that it was impressive to see that whatever the diet of the month was, it was easy to get the right types of foods and cook great meals. In other words, there is a lot of different foods available and it is not difficult to try new diets.

Tomas:

No matter what your food restrictions are, it is possible to eat delicious healthy foods.

The diets I did not do

One of the things that became clear to me, especially while editing my own log, is how many interesting diets are out there that I did not try.

For example, raw foods. If I was stuck on an island with no fire, I would try raw foods. I don't like raw meats or fish, which means that going raw is just too radical for me. But maybe one day. I'm sure my microbiome would go for a nice ride.

I also did not try he alkaline diet, which I read up on and didn't think was much different from my regular way of eating. I must admit that there is something about the alkaline diet that irks me. Physiologically, the levels of acidity in our intestinal tract are extremely variable between the stomach to the small intestine. Thinking further on this, our stomachs' acidity level is equivalent to that of a very strong acid, which could basically disintegrate soft tissue. In other words, we would be is serious trouble if the acidity of our internal digestive system was not kept precisely within the intestinal system. That said, the alkaline diet advocates whole healthy foods, and I don't eat many processed foods.

The blue-zone diet is also interesting and is purported to support a long healthy life. Mostly plant-based, the blue-zone diet is also associated with lifestyle, and includes a developed sense of family, avoiding smoking, moderate and daily physical activity, and social engagement. Although I did not do the blue-zone diet, is also not much different to my regular diet and lifestyle.

Yet another eating style that I did not do throughout this year is the ayurvedic diet. Originally from India and based on an ancient system of life (ayur) knowledge (veda), this eating style can loosely be defined as a holistic approach to health which tailors' foods and eating to three body types for maximum happiness and balance.

I love the idea of studying different ways of eating and learning about food science. Many diets, including the majority of the 12 challenges I did do, have a similar message, which is to eat whole foods. I strongly support trying something different for a couple of weeks whenever you feel like you need to reset of shock your system out.

Ketogenic, for example, is highly anti-inflammatory. If you feel like trying this diet, eat the lowest carbs possible and lots of different healthy fats for a few weeks. Make sure to incorporate plenty of above ground plants and some nuts (avoid pistachios and cashews have too many carbs) while avoiding starchy carbs and sugar.

In the end, and as I mentioned probably a million times before, it is the process and what you do on a regular basis that counts. And I don't mean that you shouldn't have a goal or a final objective, of course you should. But, in the end, the result comes, whether you like it or not.

Getting back to the 12 food challenges, there is something highly enriching about these types of experiments, whether done alone on in sequence. They reinforce the fact that we have control over our diet… we choose what we eat. And eating is the most intimate thing we do… to us and for us.

Exploring diets and trying new health-promoting foods is wonderful. I know I will try new diets in the future, but for now I need to float free and see where my food-self roams without any limits.

Overall health

As you can imagine, there were many times throughout the year where the self-imposed food limitations resulted in awkward moments with friends and family. For one thing, there was an obvious concern for my health. Often, people that care about me became awry about the potential long-term effects of some of the food challenges.

I was often questioned about whether it was a good idea to use myself as a lab rat, or to experiment with something that in the end may have long-term detrimental effects on my health. In fact, there were times that I didn't feel so great, but I consider those to be a normal part of our day to day highs and lows. I tend to avoid going to the doctor, but if I had to self-diagnose the state of my general health through all the food challenges, I would say that I have been in excellent health throughout the year.

Now looking back, I was fortunate to have chosen to do thirty days for each challenge, as it provided enough time for the body to adapt and feel the differences imposed by each eating regime. Also, the thirty day period for each challenge was not too long, and therefore turned out to be a great lesson in my capacity for physical resilience.

Except for the ketogenic diet, which had a longer adaptation period, it was impressive how quickly my body rhythms adjusted, regardless of how drastic the changes were from one challenge to the next. Either immediately or at most after a few days, my basic body functions seemed to work fine month after month.

Regular intestines, nights of undisturbed deep sleep, and mostly a regular menstrual cycle as usual. I did feel that my energy levels varied with what I ate and that this affected my capacity to meet heavy physical demands like weight training or endurance exercises. However, I am merely a recreational athlete and therefore have the luxury of opting to listen to my body and take it easy when I didn't feel that pushing it would be beneficial.

I have frequently been asked whether there were favorite challenges, or diets in which I felt better or worse. The answer is that yes, there were positive surprises which I will talk about later. But regarding my self-evaluation of overall health, I personally found the vegetarian challenges to be most difficult on my body. Although I live mostly on a plant based diet, I feel the need for animal protein.

Besides vegetarian, the ketogenic diet was the other diet that was physically demanding, especially for the first couple of weeks. There is a reason for the term "keto-flu" used to describe the tiredness and muscle pain associated with adaptation to ketosis.

That brings me to a very interesting point that repeatedly came up when I was doing the ketogenic diet. Almost everyone, including health professionals, warned me of the damage that it would do to my health and to my cholesterol levels. This motivated me to do the blood analysis after the ketogenic month as well as at the end of the challenges, with the results shown in the Table below (Table 1).

Table 1. Blood cholesterol and triglyceride levels in mg/dL

	Cholesterol (<190)	Triglycerides (<180)	LDL (<130)	HDL (>40)
May 5, 2015	254	94	150	85

Dec 2, 2016**	290	120	174	92
May 9, 2017	259	89	156	85

** blood was collected one hour after eating a bowl of full fat Greek yogurt with walnuts on day 29 of the ketogenic challenge

The total cholesterol measured in our blood is the result of the sum of low density lipoprotein (LDL), high density lipoprotein (HDL) and 1/5 of the blood triglycerides (total cholesterol = LDL + HDL + (triglycerides/5)). Although controversial, the measures of blood cholesterol are often utilized as an indication of risk for cardiac disease, with the current guidelines of acceptable levels for each lipid type shown in brackets in the top row of Table 1.

Many consider that the levels of cholesterol and triglycerides in our blood are directly proportional to the amount of fat in our diets. However, according to the scientific literature, this is just not true. In fact, the guidelines for daily cholesterol consumption as well as what is considered a healthy cholesterol level in our blood are currently under revision.

What we do know is that all of the cells in our body can synthetize cholesterol and that cholesterol is an essential structural component of our cells membranes. Furthermore, our blood cholesterol levels are more indicative of the cholesterol made by our livers (often from sugars as prime materials) than of cholesterol eaten.

Triglycerides, on the other hand, are directly deposited into our blood from the final product of fat digestion, which means that blood triglyceride levels can be directly influenced by what and when we eat. Thus, the reason why blood collection for analysis of blood cholesterol levels normally being done after a period of overnight fasting.

As you can see by my blood work, my cholesterol levels are slightly high, mostly due to very high levels of the good cholesterol HDL. Unfortunately, I hadn't planned on these food challenges going as far as they did, and don't have analysis from just prior to the first month. I do, however, have them from one year before (May 2015) and the results are generally consistent, as you can see from the final analysis done in May 2017, after all the challenges were completed.

I would like to emphasize here that the main reason that I decided to do the blood work and to show these results is to establish that eating 75% fat for a month during the ketogenic challenge did not alter my cholesterol levels! *As written in greater detail in the Ketogenic revisited section, the knowledge that fat is a healthy dietary food is currently spreading in the press, as are the negative effects of processed foods and simple carbs, such as sugar and refined flour or starch.*

It is a pity that the initial analysis from December 2nd at the end of the ketogenic month were done at the pharmacy with the quick "pricked-finger and blood drop" method. As described in detail at the end of the ketogenic chapter, the results of this practical test turned out to be completely inconsistent.

However, after a late realization of the impossibility of the results and encouragement from Patrick to repeat the test, blood collection for proper analysis was done approximately one hour after breakfast. This explains the triglyceride levels being higher than they would have been if the blood had been collected after an overnight fast. On the other hand, and to conclude this part, I was happy to see my latest measures of blood cholesterol, which were equivalent to their usual.

Food challenges and body metrics

As I mentioned at the beginning of the book, I did not choose to do food challenges with the intent to change my body shape or weight. On the other hand, although I was ok with my body, I was also aware that I had gained a few kilograms in the last few years, which I partially attributed to age and the fact that I quit smoking three and a half years ago.

Regardless, whether it was timing, the fact that I took a nutrition course, the amount of exercise I did and do, or a combination of any of these, my body did change over the year. This was most obvious to me when I took out my summer clothes a couple of weeks ago and things that I love and have hesitated to discard, even though I haven't been able to fit into for years, now fit perfectly.

I have charted my body weight in kilograms and waist circumference in cm at the end of each month, and the results are illustrated in Figure 1 below.

The one thing that I want to make very clear is that although I was happy to shed a few kilograms, there was never a point throughout the year that I avoided eating something with the purpose of losing weight. The only time that I did not eat when hungry was when it was impossible to do so because of the challenge at hand. However, I did feel the difference in my body month after month.

There was a noticeable change as the extra fat shed off and I got leaner and fitter. The challenge that incurred the biggest weight loss was the ketogenic month, but as discussed in the appropriate chapter, likely due to water loss. This is further supported by the immediate weight gain in the gluten and dairy free month afterwards.

Also interesting, is the comparable amount of weight lost in the paleo and vegan months, basically two polar opposite diets. In the end, I lost 4.7 kg over the year and 9 cm in waist circumference.

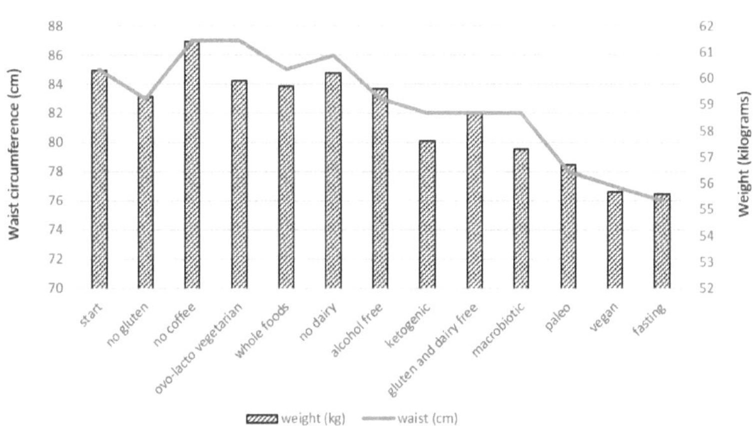

Figure 1. Body weight in kilograms (kg) and waist circumference in centimeters (cm) measured on the last day of each challenge. Over the twelve months,

there was a 9 cm decrease in waist circumference (from 85 to 76 cm), and a drop of 4.7 kg (from 60.3 to 55.6 kg).

Looking at the graph of weight and waist circumference intrigues me. I believe that the relative weight loss between diets was very much influenced by the time of the year that the challenge fell on. For example, August and December are summer holiday and Christmas months, respectively. This means that during the whole foods (August) and gluten and dairy free months (December), there were frequently festivities and breaks in routines.

Regardless of the specifics of each month, I believe that it was the staying power of sticking to the project that resulted in the narrowing down of my waist and building muscle. Unfortunately, I have dedicated very little time to moving my body in the last days as I work on this book. I find that I eat less, but am also missing the physical strength that comes from putting time into pushing my body.

Sitting here writing and editing, I feel my body softening. But that is ok, there are phases in life where balance is impossible for the priority at hand to be met. As I mentioned at the beginning of the book, it was not weight loss that incentivized me to do this. That said, I am very happy about the results. I feel better and know that I still can be and will be even better. Physically and mentally.

Back to the results as part of the process, I have no doubt that the positive outcome obtained with the body metrics can be mostly attributed to the discipline of staying with the twelve challenges. As far as exercise goes, even though I have always had periods of higher intensity physical activity, I am in general active and have been throughout the year. From the paleolithic month forward, I started incorporation the off-season training from the Ultimate Athlete Project into my weekly routine, and that may have influenced the waist circumference.

Regarding the weight loss results, I think that the challenges made me more aware of what I was eating. As species, we tend to eat a lot when food is available, and the limits forced me to eat less. One more thing that may be interesting for anyone wanting to do consecutive challenges as a weight loss method, is that the body gets used to eating less without "eating less" being the direct objective.

From the standpoint of someone that does not like to be told what to do, like me, this is a good thing.

Also, and partially due to the increased variety imposed by different limits, the gradual loss in weight may be more sustainable. Once again, I wonder how my journey with food will evolve and what I will have to say a couple of months from now, a year from now, or a decade from now. What I notice is that I eat less now than I used to. Partially, I believe that the higher fat diet that I currently eat, with a lot of nuts and seeds, keeps me feeling fuller for longer periods of time.

As a final curiosity, I did a weigh-in three weeks after the last challenge was completed, and there were no significant differences in my weight or waist in comparison to the last day of the final challenge. I weighed in at 55.8 kg and my waist was 75 cm in circumference, compared to 55.7 kg and 76 cm at the end of the fasting month, respectively. Just as I finish off the book a month and a half after the final challenge, I decided to collect one final weight/waist metrics today. Again, there have been no significant weight or waist circumference changes, with a slight loss in weight likely due to doing less exercise.

Now it is time to let go of metrics and to continue to explore with new foods and work the body. Tonight's dinner should be interesting, a vegan wholegrain salad with fresh parsley, celery and blueberries accompanied by a cashew cream sauce. The creamy sauce is very simple to do, just soak unsalted cashews in salted water overnight and then blend with some of the water to the consistency you like. I will add some olive oil, garlic and pepper to the blend to make it tasty for the salad.

The food challenges and (my) physical performance

There are always a million things related to food and sports dancing around in my mind. The biology of sports science is important and something that is very much a part of my life, especially from the perspective of training and nutrition. On one hand, I coach some incredible athletes who incorporate intensive physical activity as part of their weekly routines and who regularly have fitness objectives in their lives. And then, to add to that, the biology of full physical/mental capacity in a sustainable manner is my passion right now, occupying most of my mental space and daily working time.

I must clarify that I am by no means an expert in sports performance. I am, however, lucky to have three close friend who are; Pedro Vargas who is just finishing his PhD in sports physiology and who is coach of the national Portuguese ultimate team; Rui Pires, an expert in strength training and human joint mechanics, and; Tim Morrill, a functional performance specialist and strength and conditioning coach.

Not only are these three gurus generally available to me for endless discussions and inspiration, they are also role models for what it means to be an elite athlete, which is not necessarily a professional athlete. Through them, as well as my passion for beach ultimate, I am constantly and consistently amazed about what the human body can do.

Although I am not an elite athlete, I personally feel the need to push my body physically, and train regularly at the gym and playing beach ultimate. Regarding my own training, I am physically active. At the time of this book I was following a strength and conditioning routine from the Ultimate Athletes Project (UAP) online platform. I can proudly say that I am a consultant on nutrition for the UAP as well as for Tim Morrill Performance. Which brings me back to food, and more specifically food and athletic performance.

Before I talk about the challenges and sports, it is important to always keep in mind that physical performance is dependent on multi-factorial processes. There is no doubt that food is important, but so is sleep, emotional and intellectual stability, and training. The awareness of this and capacity to integrate is key, as is knowing that it is what you do as part of the routine that makes a difference.

Back to food and now thinking of food as the prime material, let us consider a scenario in terms of home construction. Everyone knows that a good solid house can be built with less than perfect material. Conversely, a precarious unstable house can easily be built with the best prime material. But the best house is the one that is well built with good prime material. Maintenance and upkeep are important too. So yes, eating wholesome good foods as the prime material is important, but it is nowhere near enough.

Regarding the food experiments this last year, I learnt a lot about food and became highly involved in how certain food choices influenced how I felt physically. I also read a lot, and you can find details about how I felt during each challenge as well as what the scientific literature says about their effects on athletic capacity in each specific chapter.

Looking over the entire year, I found my body slowly changing towards a more athletic body. And this, I mostly owe to the discipline of training regularly and eating whole foods rather than to one specific diet. There is also no doubt that I am right now more comfortable with a much wider circle of food choices, and that my eating has changed.

Regardless of my current objectives, I generally eat more fat and more protein, and much less carbs. I almost don't eat white bread, pasta or white rice, as these are no longer staple foods in the house. I am also very aware of my tendency for sugar-addiction, and try to think of sugar as a recreational drug and use it as such. That means it is not that bad for those times that I am demanding a lot of my body or brain, like for example simple carbs before a beach ultimate game or a healthy-sugary snack while editing this book.

The relevance and health benefits of eating a variety of plants was common to all the challenges - including husks (such as cinnamon and psyllium), seeds and various spices. Truth be told, plants generally contain chemicals which are slightly poisonous to us. However, small doses of poison from a variety of edible plants also provide amazing health benefits, including anti-inflammatory and immune stimulating properties.

For anyone, and especially for athletes who are constantly pushing their bodies beyond limits, plants and spices are a must. Try making water infusions with ginger, lemon, cinnamon, aniseed, turmeric, mixed as you like or alone. These tasty drinks are great with a little honey, hot or cold, on ice, or to take in your water bottle when training. Other great ways to use spices is to sprinkle them on simple popcorn or baked sweet potato chips. For this, spicy cayenne with a little cumin is my favorite.

As my knowledge on health expands, I become ever convinced that although there are individual truths and/or periodic truths, but there are no absolute truths. And with this I am not denying that there are strategies through diet that potentiate specific goals, such as for example, protein after training being important for muscle repair and synthesis. From a long-term perspective, nutrition must adapt to the individual athlete, respecting and adapting to changing needs.

In other words, specific goals and adaptation of nutrient strategies to the individual athlete's responses are essential. A recently published review by Burke and Hawley (Science Vol 362, page 781), entitled Swifter, higher, stronger: What's on the menu?, establishes the key role of Carbohydrates, with daily CHO intakes varying from 2 to 12 g per kilogram of body mass between athletes and training cycles.

The authors also suggest a daily protein intake target of 0.3 g per kilogram of BM high quality protein at four to six meals or snacks. particularly 1-3 hours after key training sessions and maybe a double dose before sleep. Apart from macro-nutrients, athletes can have increased requirements for certain nutrients, such as electrolytes, water, iron or risk of vitamin deficiencies.

There is no doubt that the human body is extremely adaptable. Yet, it is clear both intuitively as well as from the science literature that we should eat good wholesome foods to meet nutritional needs. Foods that represent the diverse mix of options found in nature, and preferably as close to the form they exist in nature as possible. The best is to be open minded and able to adjust to the foods available while listening to our bodies. Sounds simple, right?

In fact, adjusting to our changing needs and the foods available is the toughest part, since nothing is static and we tend to prefer quick results that don't require much thinking or decision making. I heard something the other day that stuck. Digested, it said: no one wants a vitamin pill, people want painkillers. Unfortunately, in my opinion, painkillers do not resolve anything. Not long-term, anyway.

Life generally lasts a long time and we need your bodies/brains at their best throughout. This means that it is important to keep sustainability in mind when exploring your body and pushing limits for maximal performance. Growth and improvement requires time for repair and integration. Ideally, make the time for self-care and to heal, to reflect, to fail... take time to cook and explore foods. In the end, it is all connected.

I think of this year as a year spend perfecting the food anthropologist's toolbox. Familiarity with foods is a fantastic tool for everyone, and especially for athletes who are constantly pushing their body to go beyond. The 12 challenges were a huge lesson, resulting in a large increase in the variety of food cooked at home, which in turn fed back, largely increasing the number of possible choices of what to eat. As an added bonus, positive actions towards our health often encourage more positive actions.

Balance, limits, and sustainability

I hope I don't come across as high-headed in what I'm about to write, but I often think about the sustainability of our planet and want to write a bit on this important topic. To be clear, what is written here is my perspective of things, my opinion, and by no means meant to be an absolute truth. Please keep a curious and forgiving mind while you read, and hopefully think about taking positive measures yourself.

The whole premise of this section is that we, as a species, could work much better alone and together to make this world a healthier and more balanced place to live. Our planet is ageing, and I mean us, we are ageing to live decades after retirement. At this point, our economic system can't afford the luxury of supporting so many old people. Especially if they are inactive and in increasing need of health care for many years.

The good news is that there is that humans can be active and useful to society at any age, and often almost up to until the day they die. Unfortunately, and for many complex reasons, our society does not empower the elderly. That said, each one of us can make a difference by making healthier decisions on how we live our day to day lives.

Our lifestyle choices matter on many levels, both personal and societal, as they can greatly reduce the period of morbidity (time that we are dependent on others for care) at the end of our lives. Collectively, we can make an impressive difference by individually taking small steps. And I am not talking about feeding the existing multi-billion dollar industries such as the cosmetic, and anti-aging businesses. Also, I am not referring to spending more time and/or money to find out what could possibly be wrong with each of us as individuals by doing various fancy biotech tests.

What I am talking about is the serious immediate need for individual actions, involving the incorporation of more grass-roots lifestyles. And I hate to be cliché, but more integration. We all know what we could do to better our health as well as what small steps we could take towards environmental awareness and to save our planet. The tough part is to make these measures a part o our routines.

We are a mortal species, which means aging and death are part of our process. In this vein, I think everyone can benefit from reading a book entitled "Being Mortal", written by the surgeon Atul Gawande. In this important read, the author confronts the realities of aging and dying in our modern society. From my perspective, continuing to learn and to push beyond current personal limits are part of ageing gracefully and sustainably. This means resisting the natural tendency to avoid new experiences and choosing to find comfort in routines.

This unfortunate tendency for the safe comfortable has many limiting effects on us. One of the most damaging being that we often avoid doing things we have never done, and therefore forget how pleasurable it is to learn something new. Eventually, as time passes without trying something new, or worse yet avoiding being exposed to new things, we develop a fear for new experiences. Thus, the natural age-related narrowing of our limits, such as our physical capacity for example, narrow even more.

I have no doubt of the huge societal impact that would result if we all actively avoided letting life take over to narrow our capabilities as we age. I believe that pushing ourselves and consistency is the way to contradict the decay and to lengthen capacity. Furthermore, our food, brain, body, and emotional selves are in truth one. We must not lose sight of the "whole person" while maintaining a balanced positively challenging life.

Eat well, move, sleep seven to eight hours a day, love, laugh, and think about our planet... walk when you can, buy locally grown organic foods, avoid processed, recycle. Avoid single use plastic and consumerism. If you do feel like treating yourself to something new, try second hand stores/fairs! Of course perfection does not exist, and not every day is a good day, but in the end, it is what we do as part of our routines that makes a difference.

Besides sleeping, moving is a big part of our health. Important practical guidelines are provided by a recent publication entitled Physical Activity Guidelines (PAG) for Health and Prosperity in the United States (JAMA. Published online November 12, 2018). The authors point to data showing that only 26% of men, 19% of women, and 20% of adolescents in the United States meet the PAG recommendations. This, of course, translates into a huge loss in health and a rise in health costs.

According to the PAG, "sufficient physical activity for adults is at least 150 minutes of moderate-intensity aerobic physical activity per week combined with 2 days per week of muscle-strengthening activity. For youth (6 through 17 years), recommendations include at least 60 minutes of moderate-intensity aerobic physical activity per day and 3 days per week of muscle-strengthening activity". Billions of dollars and hundreds of thousands of lives could potentially be saved if these recommendations were met, not to speak of the improvement in quality of life

The health benefits of physical activity are enormous, including reducing the risk of diseases such as obesity, type 2 diabetes, cardiovascular disease, dementia, and 8 forms of cancer (bladder, breast, colon, endometrium, esophagus, kidney, lung, and stomach). Also essential, physical activity improves sleep and therefore brain function.

In truth, we can be useful if we lead healthy productive lives. And longevity is only worthwhile with some quality, an issue often overlooked by our current healthcare system. The Global Burden of Disease database (http://www.healthdata.org/gbd) is worth perusing if you are interested in the global health issue. It provides excellent data on the burden of disease as well as years lived with disease per global region. Moreover, the compare tool (https://vizhub.healthdata.org/gbd-compare/), allows us to compare specific causes of mortality and disease across regions, age, and gender. This data is invaluable for the development of health guidelines and measures. Also, let us not forget that our lifestyle is the main influencer of our health, a lot of which is in our hands.

No matter where you are on your health journey, trying and sticking to something different is always good. Besides physical activity, trying different healthy diets is a fantastic example of a positive way to fight the resistance for change. Not only that, trying different eating modes is a great incentive to learn new recipes and to experiment with new healthy foods. Variety in what we eat is great for us and for the microorganisms that live in our gut.

In the end, the capacity to change and to stick to a plan is hugely empowering, and a fantastic exercise in discipline. Also, one small step towards health often results in a ripple effect of good health-promoting behaviors in other areas of our lives. I believe that similarly to it being the small changes in our actions that make a difference in our lives and our health, it is what we do as individuals that makes the difference in society. And it is always worth it and never too late to start.

Afterthoughts

In this afterthoughts section, written in November 2018, I am going to take the mental and literary space to widen the perspective of this book beyond the food challenges. Bear with me as I put this out there for you.

As publication of this revisited version approaches, I am feeling excited and positive. I am particularly grateful to those that sent me their thoughts and opinions. Even now, after this revision, it rests my mind to consider that changes are possible, and that this work is not final or static. Nevertheless, I have thoroughly enjoyed re-reading and revising the book. As I was telling Patrick, Sara, and Nuno, one of the owners of a favorite local restaurant, *Restaurante Sociedade* at SMUP, I believe this work has improved, and look forward to your feedback.

Also, it is unlikely that I will feel as insecure as I did the first time I published, resulting in sleepless nights every time I got a message from a friend saying their book had arrived. At this point, I have gained sufficient distance from the book to not take it so personally. Before I go off on my divagations, I think it is worth going into some overall leftover and all-encompassing feelings and opinions about the experimental year, and to tie up some loose ends. One issue that I think is important to talk about is the topic of cheating, or rather not cheating.

Besides the few unintentional slip-ups in the gluten-free month, I did not waver from doing what I said I was going to do for the rest of the year. And sticking to the diets was a huge point of honor. To be honest, I was surprised by my persistence to stick with the project as the days, weeks, and months passed. By establishing a growing sense of self-trust, this experiment turned out to be immensely empowering for me.

I also realized that I have way more will-power than I thought, and much more discipline. Or I did for this project, anyway. I have always tended to be decadent, of giving into my desires and doing what I felt like rather than what I know I should do. This journey was a fantastic lesson in discipline. Even when I seriously questioned what my intent was, or when I felt what I interpreted to be negative physical effects of certain diets, I stuck with it.

The actual order of the consecutive challenges is another point that is worth mentioning. I have often thought about whether it would have been different if the order of the diets had been different. No doubt that my perception of each of the challenges was very much influenced by the time of year as well as the immediate physical demands on me at the time. For example, macrobiotic in the dead of winter was like a warm hug on a cold day, and paleo in spring together with increased physical training was a powerful surge.

In the end, I am very happy that the order of the challenges was as it was. Furthermore, I also like that each challenge was chosen by how I felt at the time, to the point that sometimes the choice of what to do next was decided on the last day of the preceding month.

For example, I remember being very edgy during the last week on the ketogenic diet and snapping at my coach when she suggested I try paleo next. As valid as her arguments were, I felt that I needed carbs after keto and therefore chose to do a gluten and dairy free month next. I am now sure that allowing myself to choose each challenge up until day one of that challenge helped me stay motivated.

Month after month, it was great to share my experiments with my friends and family. Not only were they supportive, they were also very interested in the specifics of the diets that I was doing, how I felt, how much I liked each challenge, what I ate, etcetera. The one question that most people asked was, "which one was your favorite challenge?" To answer this and looking back on the entire year of all twelve food regimes, there were some unexpected surprises as well as lessons that will forever change the way I eat.

As is clear by the comments in each of the specific chapters, there were good and bad moments in all the challenges. But overall, I was most surprised at how much I enjoyed the paleolithic diet. Considering that I don't normally eat that much meat, it was amazing how much I liked it.

I also did not expect the way my body reacted to being vegetarian, and it made me realize that at this point in my life I need some animal protein to feel good. As far as long-term changes or take-home lessons, it is now two years later and I still eat way less carbs than I used to. I don't mean that I am eating a lot of meat, as I continue to enjoy mostly a plant based diet. Rather, the changes are mostly that I do not eat much wheat, with my starchy carbs coming mostly from nuts, legumes and whole grains.

The biggest thing that changed in my and my family's eating is the obvious increase in flexibility and variability when it comes to foods and eating styles. Whereas we used to have many "weekly repeats", such as pasta or meat and potatoes, we now vary the menu immensely, and eat differently almost every day.

The challenges also resulted in re-setting the protein: fat: carb ratio that I eat on a daily basis. At this point, the amount of starchy carbs I eat is very much associated with how much physical exercise I do in a single day. For example, I eat an almost ketogenic diet when I spend my days sitting behind the computer, and eat carbs, especially simple carbs like pasta or rice, mostly just before, during or after doing some strenuous exercise.

Don't get me wrong, I do not impose strict or even regulated rules to what I eat. Rather, adjustments seem to come naturally. For example, I have noticed that as I I crave sugar when I use my brain a lot for writing. I happily give into my cravings, ensuring it is the good stuff and in moderation. Spicy and fruity infusions are awesome, for instance, with a little natural sweetener like honey.

Then there is the question of which one of the 12 was my favorite. The answer is that there was not one favorite, in reality none was and all were. I am sure that the lessons learnt will lead down different paths as time goes by, and that this wouldn't be possible without the whole trip.

During the year, I was often asked how I could deal with having specific food limitations for 30 days without rest, wasn't it just too difficult? In truth, it became less difficult as time went by. Each day, week and month built on each other. Via the food challenges, I pushed beyond my limits physically, emotionally, as well as intellectually. No doubt that there were tough times, but the learning curve was huge and made the effort worth it.

On a more serious note, there is something I stated at the beginning of the book and that I feel I must reiterate now. The contents of this book are not meant to be taken as scientific literature, as it is by no means a science document. All the scientific discussions herein are sprinkled with my opinions and experiences. And valid as those may be, they are not "truths" but rather a compilation of my thoughts, feelings, and subjective life.

Don't get me wrong, I do believe that this can be an important document, and hope to have been capable of pleasantly sharing the science with you, the reader. I strongly suggest to anyone who wants to learn more about the science discussed here, that they look into the original literature using an appropriate search engine, such as NCBI (https://www.ncbi.nlm.nih.gov/pubmed/). Considering that we are now in the Fall of 2018, the references provided here are a good place to start.

As a health professional, I think I would have

enjoyed reading this book, and hope that other health professionals find it interesting and worth their time. Regardless of who you, the reader, are, it is important to recognize that science is always changing and evolving... which means keeping updated with the literature is key.

Ok, here we go. I believe I saved the best for last. Please be aware that what I am about to write is based exclusively on original thoughts. This is simply not the case. Rather, my mental thread is the result of extensive reading, experiencing, thinking, living, as well as a mish-mash of many others things not mentioned specifically.

The first point I would like to discuss not directly related to the practical aspects of this book is the actual process that allowed for its completion and how that process applies to us and our lives. We humans, tend to be very much result focused. Although it is the perspective of achievement or victory that mostly drives us, a result oriented mode of operation comes with a series of problems.

There is no doubt that we need objectives and/or goals, we obviously do, and ideally realistic ones. But that does not take away from the argument that there are serious downfalls to being too focused on the result. To make my point, I would like you to consider a pyramid. When on its correct side, which is the base, the pyramid is highly stable. However, turning it upside down causes it to topple. That is what I think happens when we focus on the result (the top of the pyramid), rather than the process (which starts wide at the base and slowly works itself towards the top).

I see the inverted pyramid as a huge problem in our personal, societal, political, and financial systems. Just think of the highly skewed distribution of money or power amongst us. And the few that have a lot, typically want more. Although it not my intention to discuss my political views here, there is much to be gained from the awareness of global issues affecting health and wellness. Of particular relevance is the widening health gap that occurs as a result of inequality between the world's rich and poor.

Inequality has been on the rise in most advanced economies, mostly due to factors such as globalization, technological advances, and the shift towards a service rather than a product based economy. To read more on this, it is worth reading the November 2018 issue of Scientific American, and more specifically the forum on policy and ethics.

It is now clear that inequality widens the health and wealth gap. Although poverty is bad for our health, inequality is significantly worse... In other words, our health is particularly corroded by having our noses rubbed in what we do not have. This is evident as lower rates of infant mortality, higher life expectancy, and lower obesity and homicide in economies with greater equality, which perform better overall.

The solution to this is not easy. We have collected huge amounts of data but have not been able to close the gap or even stop it from widening. Partially, this is because data collected from an unequal society reflects that inequality, and often reinforces it. To add to that, the necessary measures are not simple and require analysis on a per-case basis. Which, once again, reinforces the importance of the process.

Be it on an individual or a collective level, results are dependent on internal as well as external factors, including perseverance to not give up, patience, forgiveness of failure, and support and encouragement from others. We all need a clear vision regarding where we want to go and allowing for adjustment based on objective analysis and feedback is key.

As anyone who is knowledgeable in coaching knows, long-term objectives should be broken down into more immediate goals that are reachable. If the focus is solely on the final result, the truth is that if the result is reached, there is not enough ground work done for further construction. The base for growth is inexistent. I find it sad how much we just love the concept of a quick success, the glorified hero idea. When in truth, the result is never as simple as it seems.

Allow me to get a little repetitive in making my point about final results by reiterating why we need the process and why victory is often anti-climactic. I can clearly see at least three oversimplified scenarios which frequently happen when we focus to much on achieving a final goal, as individuals as well as in society.

Firstly, let us assume that success is reached. The goal has been successfully achieved... and then what? It is day to day that we live, and the satisfaction received by reaching a desired goal, or a win, is at best an intense but relatively short-lived pleasure. By short lived I mean that, by itself and in isolation, the win is not enough to keep us satisfied long-term.

So, to put it bluntly, the first negative scenario is the "one-trick-pony" type of success, which normally results in disaster down the line. Conversely, when a goal is reached as part of the process, it is a sustainable result, and empowers us to take another step towards the next, more ambitious, result. And thus, the process continues.

Another and second possible negative effect of being mostly result oriented is the risk of being driven by single-minded ambition and thereby not living fully and with complete clarity. As I look around and get critical about society, it saddens me to realize how many of us are obsessed by what we think we want, and then end up living a life that is not at all what we actually wished for. Or what we expected it to be, for that matter. As I think further on this, a sad phrase comes to mind: you wanted what you have and now want what you lost.

We keep forgetting that we change. When we focus on the results sole mindedly, they can end up controlling us, and it should be the other way around. We need to control what we can, imperfectly, but consistently. Moments of doubt, failure, instability, and regression, all are ok. In fact, they help us to reestablish our goals and to lucidly face what we must do, what we have the capacity to do, which is dynamic in itself.

There is yet a third and probably most common negative outcome of focusing on the result alone, and that is failure. And not just failure of achieving the goal, but failure to continue to fight for it. As I see it, this last option is most common. Many times, we give up when we don't see the results we want, or when things are not moving forward as fast as we would like. Which brings me back to our attraction for the pain-killer as opposed to the vitamin pill, a keystone of marketing strategies and exemplary of our society today.

Of course we rarely consider that giving up is failure. Nor do we consider re-scheduling the initiation of a project, or finding yet another more exciting and often impossible substitute goal to try to reach, to be a failure. But the inverse of failure, or success, takes time to build.

Celebrating each small achievement, adjusting goals based on mindful decisions, taking time to digest acquired knowledge, acceptance of ourselves and our flaws, that is what makes us balanced and happy people with balanced and happy lives. Balance... equilibrium... for us and in our lives.

Because time doesn't stand still, being balanced is a transitory states. Which brings me to another one of my favorite topics. Our need to push beyond current limits for change and growth to occur. We are all aware of "having gone too far", be it physically, mentally, verbally, emotionally, or in any other sector of our lives. There is a point at which we go beyond what we are comfortable with, we have inevitably overstepped our limits.

Sometimes, we can even cause damage and lose some serious ground by going too far beyond. But mostly, this overstepping of our limits is internal and allows us to establish new limits. Expanding our comfort zones and establishing new limits can therefore be positive, and permits us to set new and more challenging goals, which is a needed aspect of sustainably,.

It's amazing how much we are at the mercy of our perception. Our mind and the mind of our mind and our tendency to feed back into what we already believe generally rules us. How we think and how we process our perception affects our actions, and our actions affect how we think. And not necessarily in that order. That is why challenging ourselves gives us self-trust and strength to do more.

Think of this in terms of travel, and how we feel about being in a completely strange new place. Is it a good or a bad sensation? If approached from a traveler's mind that wants to explore and learn new cultures, it is a very positive enriching experience. However, being in a completely foreign place can also be scary, bringing up strong feelings of insecurity, and loneliness.

How we perceive change is key. And experiencing change itself, succeeding at managing it and learning from it, gives us the confidence and desire to explore a little further. In this case, the journey was a self-imposed food journey. Momentum was gained as comfort zones were expanded and goals were met, which resulted in my desire to continue.

Although this journey is definitely about food, it is not exclusively about food. Like everything else in our lives, one sector trickles into another and so on and so forth. We all need to have projects. We thrive from the learning, planning, anticipation, interest, novelty, and fight. In the end, the food challenges turned out to be a fantastic project. Especially considering that the one thing that we can control is what we put, or not put, in our mouths.

Just like there are no absolute truths, some of the common "wisdom sayings" out there also irk me. For example, I just saw one today that stated, "You have everything in you to deal with whatever challenges life throws at you". If that is the case, then why are there so many unhappy and unbalanced people? Crumbling with the weight of life, in a society that does not accept or empower aging or death although it is an integral part of life?

All of us can gain a lot by us taking control of what we can control. Another saying, commonly used to empower people, is "You are in control of your life!" Without some clarification, this one also irritates me, as it forgets to consider inevitable and unpredictable life happenings that are completely external to our control. In fact, there is a reason why we need some form personal spirituality. For me, this translates into trying to not make decisions based on avoiding pain, and learning to recognize and accept the things that I cannot control, to release these from my active involvement, and to trust in the future. As balanced as that sounds, it is not always easy.

The end is here, and I would like to end in my typical optimistic fashion. A couple of days ago at the supermarket, I saw a Portuguese novel by Helena Sacadura Cabral, which the title loosely translated into: I like to like. I stared at the title and for some reason it resonated with me, and made me think how much I like to like my life, my family, my friends, what I do. And that this "liking to like" is very different from simply liking those same fundamental parts of my life, which I also avidly do.

Thinking further on this, I believe that liking to like is something we can all work on by consciously being aware of the pleasures in life. The truth is we are largely in control of what we do and as discussed earlier, our actions are an integral part of the feedback loop that formulates what we think, which in turn empowers what we do.

From a concrete and practical perspective, it is the actions that we take in our daily lives that forge our paths. Our actions and their associated mental processes are what give us the confidence in ourselves to go sustainably beyond our current comfort zones and to be happy and balanced. And, as I mentioned before, nothing human is simple. Be it food, physical exercise, learning or teaching a new skill, travel, or any other action that results in enriching change, taking action empowers us to go further in other areas of life. And that, for our integral minds/bodies as well as for our planet, is always worth it.

About the author

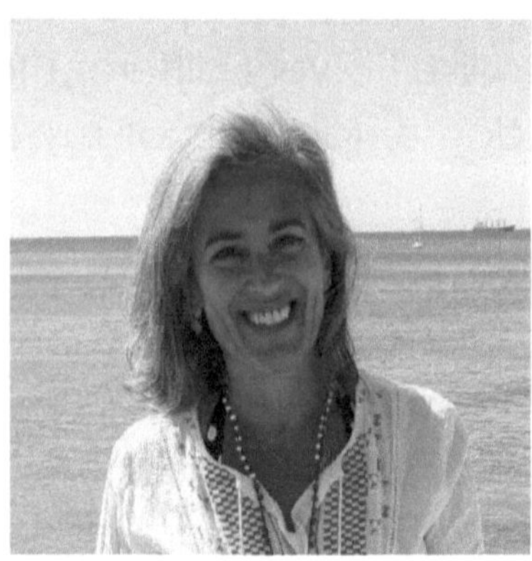

Sofia lives in a small sea-side village just outside Lisbon, the capital of Portugal. She is currently a health coach with clients from all over the world and is involved in research projects at the University of Lisbon. "The Food Anthropologist... a one year journey through food challenges", now in its revised form, was Sofia's first book.

With a PhD in biology/genetics (York University, Toronto, Canada), a long-term research background, and a health coach certificate (Institute for Integrative Nutrition, New York, USA), Sofia is highly interested in food as the building blocks of our bodies and brains, and the effects of our behavior on our physical and mental health. For more information about the author, please read on or check out Sofia's website at www.besthealth.life.

More about the author (me)

My name is Sofia, I am fifty-three years old and was born and lived in Lisbon Portugal for the first decade of life. In 1975, my family and I moved to Canada (mostly Toronto) because of the revolution in Portugal in 1974. In the mid-nineties and after living twenty years in Canada, I moved back to Portugal with my Dutch husband Patrick, who I met in graduate school in Toronto and to whom I am married to since 1993.

We got married so he didn't have to go back to Holland when his student visa expired after finishing his masters in organic chemistry. I never thought I would be into a long-term relationship, but serendipity was on my side at that decision point.

Except for a couple of years in San Francisco in 1999 and 2000, we have been living close to Lisbon in a beautiful small town on the ocean fifteen kilometers west of Lisbon for more than two decades. Also, the math says that I am married for almost twenty-four years to Patrick and living together for more than a quarter of a century.

Luckily for me, he is an amazing man who is my partner, best friend, lover, beach ultimate team mate, techie, and whatever else I need him to be. I hope to be the same for him. We also have two kids, Sara and Tomas, who we both adore infinitely. No, things are not always perfect, and there are some tough moments and phases. But overall, my immediate family of four provides me with an enriching and loving home environment where we all allow each other to fly while feeling unconditional love.

Our social life is reasonably rich, with a wide circle of friends such as work and school friends, friends from disc and family friends, living on many corners of the globe as well as close by. We also live within a few kilometers of many members of my family, who I collectively and individually care about immensely, and even if I am not necessarily involved in their daily lives, learn continuously from.

My mom is the third daughter of a large and close family, so there are frequently family celebrations. I could write extensively about the complex and wonderful relationships with my parents, brothers, step-mom, ex step-dad and sibs, cousins, friends and so on and so forth.

As far as my education, I have a hard-core science background. When I started university in Toronto Canada, I wanted to be a doctor. After a few years as a biology and chemistry undergraduate student, I fell in love with research and fundamental science during first and second year summer jobs getting paid to do research in the laboratories of the biology department.

In 1995, I completed a PhD at York University in Toronto, which was focused on behavior genetics of complex feeding behavior and had a strong component of molecular and neuro-biology. After that, I moved to Lisbon and spent two decades as a post-doc or research fellow doing research, orienting students, teaching, and basically focusing on fundamental science.

My first post-doctorate was at the Faculty of medicine in Lisbon University studying early embryonic development. Since the early 2000s, I have been doing research at the Instituto Superior de Agronomia where my interests widened to include functional genetics of crop plants. I am still involved in research and continue to dedicate some of my time to projects, meetings and hard-core science publications, but my full-time job since January 2016 is as a health coach.

There are many reasons why my life changed from that of being a full-time scientist and researcher to that of being a health coach who also does science. For one thing, due to current economics and world politics, or perhaps increasing awareness of these issues as my years advance, my passion for fundamental science was slowly surpassed by the desire to make a more practical difference in the world.

Luckily and at a friend's suggestion while in Abu Dhabi in the spring of 2015, I embarked on a one year health coach training program at the Institute for Integrative Nutrition in New York. I loved the course. It provided an ideal integrated approach to health, a comprehensive and highly practical coaching curriculum, and plenty of intelligence and additional resources to inspire me to study further.

To sum up this part quickly, I will conclude that I have no doubt that being a health coach is what I am meant to do right now. I take a very scientific approach to coaching my clients, and believe that knowledge is power when it comes to our biology. Such a complex issue. I am a strong advocate of the complete integration between our body and mind, they are in truth one whole. Which, by the way, is the origin of the word health, whole. Needless to say, the whole of health is my passion right now. If you want to know more about my education or what I do, feel free to check out my website (www.besthealth.life) or Facebook page (https://www.facebook.com/besthealthbestlife/).

There is one more thing that I must mention very quickly to sum up this part "all about me". I am highly interested in athletic performance and sports, and the concept of sustainably pushing our bodies beyond their current limits. Although I am personally not a sports expert, I have close friends that I consider sports gurus who are critical in my learning process and provide me with great discussion and criticism. Also, I provide consulting in nutrition and coaching to Ultimate frisbee athletes and, have followed various comprehensive periodical training plans.

As discussed in the body of the book, moving our bodies is key. As I get older, I know that it is not worth trying to concentrate when I sit for too long. For my brain to work, I need to move, plain and simple. When my kids tell me they are having difficulties studying, I often tell them to go for a walk, or do some exercise for10 minutes. I know that flexibility, endurance and strength are key for a good life, and I try to incorporate time for all three regularly. Personally, I love to push my body by playing sports with friends, and still practice beach ultimate regularly. Finding balance is key, coupled with cherishing the wonders of life.